Stroke FORWARD

How to Become Your Own Healthcare Advocate . . . One Step at a Time

MARCIA MORAN

ISBN: 978-1-7332587-0-8

Library of Congress Control Number: 2019910396

Printed in Centreville, Virginia, USA by Moran Consulting, LLC

Photo Credits: Jessica Wallach, Marianne Meadows, and Marcia Moran

Disclaimer

The publisher has strived to be as accurate and complete as possible in the creation of this book.

This book is not intended for use as a source of legal, health, or medical advice. All readers are advised to seek the services of competent professionals in legal, health, or medical fields.

The advice and strategies found within may not be suitable for every situation. This work is sold with the understanding that neither the author nor the publisher is held responsible for the results accrued from the advice in this book. Readers are cautioned to rely on their own judgment about their individual circumstances and to act accordingly.

While all attempts have been made to verify information provided for this publication, the publisher assumes no responsibility for errors, omissions, or contrary interpretation of the subject matter herein. Any perceived slights of specific persons, peoples, or organizations are unintended.

For more information, visit www.StrokeForward.com.

Toastmasters International® and all other Toastmasters International trademarks and copyrights are the sole property of Toastmasters International. This book is the opinion of the author and is independent of Toastmasters International. It is not authorized by, endorsed by, sponsored by, affiliated with, or otherwise approved by Toastmasters International. To learn more about Toastmasters International, visit www.Toastmasters.org.

DEDICATION

To all of the people who have suffered from a traumatic brain injury and their caregivers. Know that you are not alone. Very few people understand the process of becoming your own advocate, of developing self-determination and the ability to choose and make decisions on your own after a life-altering medical event.

I didn't think about healthcare advocacy as I struggled along my journey, but looking back, the actions my husband, Jim, took on my behalf made him my advocate in the hospital and after my release. He asked the important questions, and spoke up for me so I could get both the care and resources I needed while I recovered. Later, he struggled while I learned to take responsibility back because I needed to become my own advocate. I wanted to become an independent person again. I'll let you know a little secret. I was often scared. But I still moved forward.

Hopefully you will find comfort in knowing that all brain injury survivors are scared sometimes. We prevail because we choose to take a chance and keep moving forward.

TABLE OF CONTENTS

INTRODUCTION

I've always been a storyteller. Finding the right words to describe an experience—whether mine or someone else's—has always been second nature. Storytelling is why I founded my company, Performance Architect, in 2012. It gave me an outlet for my creativity as I focused on leadership, human behavior, and exceptional performance stories that served to fuel others' achievements.

I had grown the company to where I would garner a nice income in 2014. Life was looking pretty sweet. Life outside of work was great as well. I was physically active, spending time jogging, kayaking, or hiking with Jim and enjoying the outdoors at our lake house. When I wasn't moving, I was painting, another creative outlet.

Six birds, one cat, one husband, and a business. I had it all. And then I experienced the unexpected: I had a stroke.

Many people look at a stroke as a terrible thing. I don't. Yes, it changed my life. It has been a challenge to recover from the stroke that assaulted my brain and body. It has also given me a sense of belonging that I never believed was possible.

It became clear early on that someone needed to be my advocate. My husband took on that role after my stroke. He became my voice and the keeper of my health information. He learned quickly that he also had to be my protector, watching everything that the nursing staff and others did for, and to, me. He was also responsible for carefully weighing the information my healthcare providers told me, while I struggled to remember what their flood of words meant. I could talk but communicating clearly wasn't feasible. As if that wasn't enough, we learned the hard way that Jim needed to monitor food from the hospital's kitchen. I might've choked to death if it wasn't pureed.

Insurance wasn't a worry for us like it is for so many. We were lucky because we had a policy that worked well. It paid for the tests and took care of everything I needed so Jim didn't have to think about it.

What we didn't have was a healthcare directive that would have informed the hospital of my wishes regarding a variety of medical possibilities. For example, what if I had needed to be resuscitated? I didn't have a document that would have told the hospital personnel whether I wanted this option or not. The staff didn't know what I wanted, and we didn't have anything in writing. While everything worked out fine for me, the lack of a healthcare directive could be a glaring omission for someone else.

In the absence of another person to be your advocate, a healthcare directive alerts the staff to your wishes. They're legally bound by this signed, notarized document. Yes, it costs money for an attorney to draw it up, but it can save genuine heartache later.* Note: DNR rules vary by state. Please consult an attorney.

I survived my hospital experience. Then, I had to learn how to become my own advocate and reclaim my independence. Jim did an exemplary job of getting me to the point where I felt I could be doing things on my own. Now, it was my turn to take the reins of my care and healing.

Telling my story wouldn't be complete without adding the voices of those who cared for and about me. As you read, you'll see headings that indicate a different "Perspective." Those who graciously lent their observations and feelings round out my narrative. I'm incredibly grateful to all who contributed to my healing and this book.

If you are a caregiver who has been thrust into guarding over someone, hopefully you will pick up some tips and insights as you hear from other people in my life who were plunged into the same position very suddenly.

If you are someone who is a patient with a serious brain injury, this book is for you. From my story, you will see that some of the struggles you have, I have also faced. I've shared key learnings that you can add to your toolbox and use to expand upon as you also get better.

Every brain injury is different, so please feel free to skip around so you focus on those areas that are specific to you. Each chapter ends with a section called **Take Action**. These are foundations I and my caregivers used on our way to recovery.

I believe in giving back. *Ten percent of the profits from this book are donated to Brain Injury Services so they can continue their critical work.*

A Special Gift from Marcia

Now that you have your copy of *Stroke* **FORWARD,** you are on your way to overcoming the hurdles of dealing with a brain injury. Plus, you'll receive insights from my story about how we "took action" so you can start applying the lessons that we had to learn on the fly and many times, the hard way.

There's so much confusing information out there about strokes and brain injuries. I learned from reading a number of books, blog posts, and videos as I struggled to find out how to get "whole." The wisdom gained along the way is shared here in the hope it will help you. When you finish this book, you'll be armed with more information to keep moving forward. With hard work and perseverance to build new neuropathways, you can make a difference in your life regardless of how the stroke impacted you.

I've created a special bonus gift, just for you. It's your *Stroke Forward Toolkit*, which is a compilation of different exercise videos, my recommended resource list, and a guide with my favorite lessons, the ones that had the greatest impact in my recovery. While the exercise videos are offered for sale, you can claim them (and the rest of the goodies) for free here: **https://www.StrokeForward.com/bookbonus**. As an additional bonus, you will receive more tips and information to help you on this journey. You may, of course, unsubscribe at any time.

The sooner you discover how to gain strength and confidence and learn ways to overcome the heartbreak, the better your chances for gaining your life back. It is, after all, a numbers game. Although you can get better every day, week, month, or even years later, the sooner you start the journey, the more progress you will make.

I'm in your corner. Let me know if I can help further.

Here's to being a thriving stroke survivor!

All my best,

Marcia

Chapter 1

SURVIVING THE UNEXPECTED

My life permanently changed on March 30, 2014.

When I awoke on that Sunday, I felt "off" in a way I'd never experienced before. I also remembered I had coffee scheduled with my friend Rochele Kadish later that morning, but based on how I was feeling, I knew I wouldn't be able to keep our date. I sat up in bed and picked up my mobile phone to text her. No matter how hard I tried, something kept jumbling the message. Finally, I gave up. I decided to get some more sleep. I'd text her later.

As I laid back down, I felt an intense throbbing in my head. I turned onto my left side. The pain exploded with a bang! I'd never experienced anything so horrible. I tried but failed to change positions; I was too weak. At that point, I wasn't thinking about my mother's death from an aneurysm. Despite my discomfort, I drifted off.

When I awoke the second time, my right side was completely limp. I knew I was in real trouble. I also knew that if I didn't get up at that moment, I might not wake up a third time. I could hear the TV downstairs that Jim, my husband, was watching. I just needed to get to him! I felt an adrenaline rush. With effort, I maneuvered my body toward the edge of the bed. Once there, gravity took over and I landed on the floor. I sized up the distance between where I was and the door. Adrenaline again flooded my veins as I dragged myself across the carpet. Using the strength of my left side to pull me along, I yanked myself inch by painful inch toward the door.

When I reached the fully shut door, it seemed as though it was taunting me. I stared up at the handle, knowing that I'd have to sit up to grip it. I lay there for a while, trying to catch my breath. I knew it would be a challenge to coordinate my half-working body so that I could grab the handle. I finally gave it a whirl. After several tries, I successfully grabbed the handle and the latch gave way. Success! The door was barely open, but that was all I needed. Achieving this feat took far too much energy. It was time for another rest. A few minutes later, I found the strength to pull the door open just wide enough for me to crawl into the hallway.

Since the surface changed from carpet to hardwood, I thought it would be easier to move along the hallway, but it wasn't. My strength was waning. Slowly, I moved closer to the stairs. By now, I was exhausted. Moving even a little bit took every ounce of my strength. Inevitably, I ran out of gas; I couldn't move. I kept thinking that Jim would have to come up for a soda at some point.

I don't know what it was, but something near me suddenly fell with a loud *crash*! Jim rushed upstairs and knelt by my side. "Marcia?" he said. "Are you all right? Can you talk to me?"

I looked at him. I remember thinking, *This is interesting. I can't speak.* He grabbed his phone and called 911. I felt a measure of relief; an ambulance was coming. Other than a quick look into the bedroom, Jim stayed by me while we waited for the paramedics. We were both frightened. Neither of us knew what would happen to me.

The paramedics arrived quickly. The first question they asked was at what time I'd had the stroke. Jim didn't know, and I couldn't respond.

I remember thinking, *Your guess is as good as mine. I didn't know what time I woke up and tried to text Rochele.* They could have looked at my phone if someone, besides me, had known that I had tried to text her. Unfortunately, the stroke had occurred while I slept. I didn't know how long I was out during my second sleeping period, nor did I know how long it took me to get from the bed to the hallway stairs. I was clueless.

Their question was critical because our answer would dictate their next care decision—whether to administer tPA or not.

"In 1995, an NIH-funded clinical trial established the first (and only) FDA-approved treatment for acute ischemic stroke. The drug tPA (tissue plasminogen activator), currently approved for delivery within 3 hours of stroke symptoms, reduces the risk of disability and maximizes the potential for patient recovery."[1]

A tPA, or tissue plasminogen activator, was out of the question because we didn't know when the stroke occurred. According to the National Institute of Neurological Disorders and Stroke, if a patient is outside of the three-hour window, tPA isn't reasonable (at the time of the stroke). Tissue death due to inadequate blood supply would mean no viable brain tissue would be left in the affected area. The paramedics made the right choice for me that day.

At least I had worn clothes to bed the night before, so I didn't have to wonder what the paramedics thought of me. They strapped me into the carrier and we left the house. They were discussing where to take me. Hope Hospital was closer at only a little over four miles; however, Greensboro Hospital had a reputation for excellent stroke care but was nearly six miles farther. We headed toward Greensboro, and I slid into unconsciousness.

JIM'S PERSPECTIVE

I woke up on March 30, 2014, around 6:00 a.m. or so, and headed downstairs so as not to wake Marcia, who typically liked to sleep in on the weekends. I frequently think about how things might have been different if I'd slept in that morning, too. I might have helped minimize the effects of the stroke for her by catching it sooner or, at a minimum, saved her from the struggle just to get to me. Thinking about her having to crawl across the floor, pulling herself along an inch at a time, still makes me sick to my stomach.

That morning, I sat watching my weekend sports with the sound low, so I didn't wake Marcia. I'm glad I did. Otherwise, I may not have heard the various sounds coming from upstairs. The first thing I remember hearing was Marcia getting out of bed. At least, I believe that may have been the correct event. For some time after, I heard her rustling around in the bedroom. I now know these sounds must have been her efforts to make her way across the floor, opening the door, and moving into the hallway. After that, I didn't hear anything. Marcia must have been inching her way down the hallway at that time.

To this day, we still don't know what fell to the floor upstairs. It sounded loud enough that I believed Marcia would need help cleaning up a mess or righting whatever had fallen. Regardless, I made my way upstairs to see what had happened. When I reached halfway up the second set of stairs from the split-level landing, I stopped. There, lying on the floor only a few feet from the stairs, was Marcia.

As I climbed the few remaining stairs, I had a fleeting thought about Marcia's chronic back problems. I thought the noise I heard was her falling. So, although it's the first thing anyone always asks and can be a foolish thing to say, I asked, "Are you all right?" If it had been her back, she would've been able to answer. Marcia said nothing. She simply peered up at me with a look I'd never seen from her before. Her look was one of combined fear and confusion.

Since she didn't reply to my first question, I moved to the next obvious question, "Can you talk?" Again, she only looked up at me. I knew then that it wasn't her back but something much more serious. But what? Regardless, the next thing I said was not a question, but a statement, "I'm calling 911." Much to my surprise, she actually gave me a slight nod.

After making the 911 call with a bit of a shaky voice, I walked around upstairs to see what may have happened. Based on some things I saw, I deduced that Marcia might have been on the toilet when the event occurred. The loud thud I heard could've been her falling from the stool. If this had been the case, then the stroke would've occurred within the last half hour and within an hour of when the paramedics arrived. After my brief investigation, I sat with Marcia to wait for the paramedics.

They arrived quickly. After entering the house, two tended to Marcia, while a third asked me questions. With one look at Marcia, they all knew what had happened. I still didn't know. I can still remember how shocked I felt when one of the paramedics said the word "Stroke." They wanted to know if I knew what had happened. I explained the sounds I heard and my thoughts on the result. In response to my assumptions, he asked if I knew for sure whether she'd had the stroke within the last three hours. Since I couldn't be sure, they didn't give her the tPA that would've helped minimize the stroke's effects. They made the right call because the stroke likely occurred more than three hours before.

As they placed Marcia on a gurney, the third paramedic said that they would be taking her to Greensboro Hospital. I immediately asked why they weren't going to the Hope Hospital, which was half the distance. The paramedic explained Greensboro's expertise in assisting stroke patients, so I agreed. He also told me to follow them to the hospital, but to drive at a normal pace. They didn't want me to get into an accident trying to hurry to the hospital. I was assured that they would take good care of Marcia.

ROCHELE'S PERSPECTIVE

"I am a trailblazer." Those were Marcia's first words when she introduced herself to our 2012 *Well-Being Foundations of Personal Transformation Cohort.* "I am a trailblazer" reverberated in my head. I was awed at her strength and confidence! I wanted to be her friend. Over the next year plus, a great friendship blossomed. We shared many common interests: kayaking, knitting, and running. And, our husbands got along, too!

Marcia and I had a breakfast date on March 30, 2014. I arrived, got us a table, and waited. A few minutes' wait is normal. When she didn't show up, I knew something was wrong. I left multiple text messages that were met with silence. I went home thinking something must have happened, and I'd hear a good story later. The next morning, after not hearing anything, I panicked. My husband and I drove to her house. No one was home. We looked all around; it was quiet. We saw a neighbor and questioned him. Did he know anything? He mentioned an ambulance had been at their home the previous morning.

Jim called that evening and he sounded like he was beside himself. In a shaky voice, he said, "Marcia had a stroke." The word *stroke* ran through my body all the way to my toes. My heart sank. I was so sad for Marcia and Jim. I was also sad for me. I wondered about our friendship. We had so many things planned. I knew things would be different and didn't know what lay ahead. The only thing I was sure of, I would do anything to support Marcia trail blaze this unforeseen path.

Well, a blog on *New York Times* website, suggests that confused or rambling thoughts that come up in speech, often common in stroke, can also be indicated via text messages.[2]

TAKE ACTION

Decide to live.

I had a decision to make the second time I awoke:

- Take Action: Get out of bed and do everything I could to get help

- Do Nothing: Accept what had happened and give up

I chose to *take action* and made my way down the hall, despite the pain. That decision clearly defined who I was, the "me" that I never really knew existed. But, more importantly, that decision defined who I'd become from that point on.

Strokes, per the National Heart, Lung, and Blood Institute, occur for two reasons:

- "An ischemic stroke occurs if an artery that supplies oxygen-rich blood to the brain becomes blocked. Blood clots often cause the blockages that lead to ischemic strokes."

- "A hemorrhagic stroke occurs if an artery in the brain leaks blood or ruptures (breaks open). The pressure from the leaked blood damages brain cells. High blood pressure and aneurysms are examples of conditions that can cause hemorrhagic strokes. (Aneurysms are balloon-like bulges in an artery that can stretch and burst.)"[3]

Similarly, some patients have a "mini-stroke," or a transient ischemic attack (TIA). Blood flow to the brain is stopped briefly. Brain cells continue to live with a TIA, and damage is reversible.

Chapter 2

BECOMING A PATIENT

Jim recounts our welcome at the hospital. I was unconscious, and he had to deal with the admitting staff.

JIM'S PERSPECTIVE

I went to the emergency room when I arrived at the hospital. From there, they directed me to Marcia's room. When I arrived, the doctors were still examining and stabilizing her. No sooner had I walked into the room when at least three people began inundating me with questions. One person wanted to know what had happened and needed specific information about Marcia. As I tried to answer, the others spoke up with different questions. It was too much. As a result of everything that had happened in the last hour or so, and the barrage of questions, I began to lose consciousness. Oddly calm, I sat down in a nearby chair, held up my hand, and said to everyone prodding me for information, "Please give me a moment; I'm blacking out."

I'm sure if I'd have completely blacked out, they would've been more concerned. They waited patiently until my head was clear again. Then, again in an oddly tranquil manner, I instructed them, "Please, one at a time." Finally, using the information I provided, plus what they were able to acquire from Marcia's online medical records from her general practitioner, they were able to focus on getting Marcia stabilized and settled in for her stay.

ADMISSION DIAGNOSIS

While I "slept," they took me in for tests. I was admitted with a diagnosis of an "acute stroke." This is a common diagnosis because most strokes start abruptly and deteriorate swiftly. My diagnosis was determined by Magnetic Resonance Imaging (MRI). It showed an acute left middle cerebral artery involving the left cerebral cortex in the Sylvian fissure region and the left lentiform nucleus and left caudate. Translated, this means I had a left hemisphere stroke, causing right-sided paralysis from my toes to my face. I was also experiencing aphasia, an inability to process language because the blood stopped flowing through a certain portion of the left side of my brain. Another finding confirmed the soundness of the paramedic's decision not to administer tPA. While my stroke was considered ischemic, I would have had a second, post-stroke bleed. Had they given me tPA, the consequences would have been devastating.

How I came to be in the emergency room that day may have had roots in the recent past. Two weeks before my stroke, I developed really high blood pressure after eating popcorn at the movies. I knew all that salt wasn't good for me, so I took my blood pressure after arriving home. I was shocked and scared when my blood pressure reading came out so high. When it didn't go down over time, I asked Jim to take me to the hospital. The staff didn't run any tests, and I was sent home without drugs. Two weeks later, the entire carotid artery severed, blocking blood flow to part of my brain. I believe that one layer of my artery wall tore first, and then the other two sections fragmented over time. No one knows for sure, but I believe that if it had been a weekday and Jim hadn't been home, I would've died on the hallway floor.

According to MedLink Neurology, bleeding post-ischemic stroke can be a misinterpreted circumstance. With tPA use becoming more common for strokes (used for strokes that occur under three to four and one-half hours) and the enhanced depiction by advanced MRI, post-stroke bleeds can be forecasted with greater accuracy.[4]

The doctors ran eleven different tests on me. I remember being rolled down for one Computed Tomography (CT) scan, but I honestly don't remember any of the others because I was unconscious.

AWAKE AND CURIOUS

When I awoke, Jim was sitting by my bed in the emergency room. *Look at that*, I thought. *Somebody dressed me in a hospital gown.* Peering around, I could see that someone had also stuck a needle in my arm. It's odd, but for someone afraid of needles, it didn't bother me. The monitors made a noise as I stared up at Jim. He was there. That was enough. I went back to sleep.

JIM'S PERSPECTIVE

Encouraging the stroke survivor to use the affected body parts as soon as possible, and re-establishing normal patterns are essential to stroke recovery.

That evening, a physical therapist came to take Marcia for a walk. She wrapped a harness around Marcia's waist and, holding the harness tightly, led her around the nurses station. Marcia did an excellent job, which showed for the first time how well she would do in her overall recovery.

THERAPY BEGINNINGS

I do remember that a physical therapist suggested that we try walking around the nurses station. I had hemiparesis by this point. I was weak down the right side of my body. Jim held my hand as I carefully got out of bed. The smell of hospital disinfectant wafted over to me. I don't know why, but it reminds me of having too much ozone in the air.

While Jim is full of praise as to how well I did on that afternoon romp, I thought I was lurching rather than walking. My right side had regained some mobility, but not much. I felt like I was in the Mel Brooks movie, *Young Frankenstein*. The scene that came to mind? Gene Wilder, who plays Dr. Frankenstein, grabs the cane from Igor and clomps down the stairs to "walk this way" as Igor had done. I didn't have Igor's hump on my back, but my right foot hiked to the outside as it clomped along.

The physical therapist held me up while I walked. Without her support, I likely would have fallen. I willed myself to stay upright and make progress toward my bed. Ever so sluggishly, we made our way around the nurses station with the physical therapist encouraging me every few feet. When we got back to my bed, I was ecstatic! I made it all the way around the nurses station without falling or needing to stop for a rest. Once the physical therapist took the harness off, I lay down. I fell asleep almost immediately.

JIM'S PERSPECTIVE

I stayed as late as they would allow that first night, but eventually, I went home. I really don't remember much about that night, other than making several phone calls to family and friends. I limited the number of friends I called and asked each to help communicate Marcia's situation to the various groups of friends we had. Doing this kept me from being inundated with phone calls and allowed me to focus on Marcia. I did choke up a couple of times talking with people about what happened. Yet, fear hadn't set in.

What I did after the phone calls is a blur. I think I finally ate something and then prepared to go to bed. I was running strictly on autopilot. The only thing I made sure to do was to set the alarm so that I could be at the hospital as early as possible the next morning. I vaguely remember pondering the day's events, as well as the major life changes that would soon follow. Despite these thoughts, my exhaustion led me to quickly fall asleep.

DALE'S PERSPECTIVE

Marcia is the baby of our family. I'm her sister, Dale, and am eight years older than her. We have a brother, Keith, who's five years older than Marcia. We're spread out across the country. Marcia lives on the East Coast, Keith in the Midwest, and I live on the West Coast. Keith and his wife, Jeanne, provided our parents with the only grandchildren, Shawn and Scott, who both live close to me. Shawn and his wife, Christy, have two young children, Parker and Carson. Except for Marcia and Jim, the whole family was gathered at Shawn and Christy's in Western Washington on the same day Marcia had her stroke.

We had a wonderful time being together, eating dinner, and watching Carson smear chocolate cake on his face. We tried calling Marcia and Jim, but there was no answer, so we left a message. We weren't concerned because they have a busy life, and we just thought they were out doing something.

It wasn't until we got home late that evening that we found out something was terribly wrong. When my husband, Joel, said that Jim was on the phone, I thought it was odd. Marcia is always the one who called me, not Jim. He usually went to bed early because he had to get up early for work.

As soon as Jim started speaking, I knew the news wasn't good. "Marcia has had a stroke," Jim said. She was alive. That was good.

Our family has a history of strokes. Our grandmother died from a stroke, and our mother died from a brain aneurysm. We knew it was serious.

The difference between a stroke, which is an event, and an aneurysm, which is a condition, can be confusing according to FlintRehab. A hemorrhagic stroke occurs when an artery ruptures and deprives the brain of blood. An aneurysm is a fragile, bulging weakness on the surface of a brain artery. An aneurysm often remains undetected until it ruptures, which results in a hemorrhagic stroke.[5]

For now, Marcia was stable, and Jim had gone home to get some rest. I wasn't sure he'd be able to sleep. I chose to take it as a good sign that the hospital had sent him home. If she'd been in immediate, mortal danger, they would have kept him at the hospital. There would be tests in the morning, and Jim would update me when he knew the results. I made sure he had my phone number at work.

Jim asked if I'd tell my brother and the rest of our family the news. He wasn't up to making another call. They were still all together at Shawn and Christy's, so I had only one call to make. It wasn't easy. All I could do was pass what little information I had. I realized I didn't even know what hospital she was in. I told Keith that I'd let them know where she was as soon as I heard from Jim.

It was a long night with little sleep. Keith told me later that he had hardly slept as well. We were all fearing the worst but hoping for the best. Since I wasn't sleeping, I went to work early. I'm a CPA, and it was only two weeks before the April 15 tax filing deadline. I knew I'd be making a cross-country trip and decided to start putting client tax returns on an extension, so I could clear my desk as much as possible. I was busy, but I found that waiting for the phone to ring seemed to make time drag. I tried not to worry, but kept wondering why Jim hadn't called; what was taking so long, and would the news be good or bad?

WAS IT FAMILY OR FATE?

I've often thought about what happened that Sunday. Stroke just didn't make sense for someone as fit as I was. My cholesterol was in the normal range. I weighed 130 pounds. I exercised regularly. Yet, I had a spontaneous stroke, which means that there was no precursor to it. I had a stroke because . . . I had a stroke. That's the scary thing. It can happen to anyone. In fact, according to Deane, et al. in a report on MDedge | Emergency Medicine site, internal carotid artery dissections (ICAD), spontaneous strokes, account for only one to two percent of all strokes in the United States. While that represents between eighteen to thirty-six people experiencing a spontaneous stroke every day, the statistics are even higher when the age range is narrowed. "It is responsible for ten to twenty-five percent of strokes in young and middle-aged adults. The peak incidence for ICAD is in the fifth decade, and it affects men and women equally."[6]

I was caught completely off guard.

A NOTE FROM MARCIA

One to two percent seems reasonable among all strokes until the ICAD happens to you and you calculate it out on an annual, daily, and hourly basis. If 795,000 strokes occur in the United States every year, and 140,000 people die, then there are 655,000 who need some sort of therapy. One to two percent of 655,000 patients equals 6,550 to

13,100 people who have an ICAD stroke annually, which means that 18 to 36 people have one every single day, and up to 1.5 per hour.

JIM'S PERSPECTIVE

Marcia was already awake when I arrived the next morning. She could barely speak. However, she was able to ask about my work. I happened to have the day off, but I told her not to worry about work and to focus on getting better. One of the calls I had made the previous night was to my boss, who gave me as much time off as I needed to take care of Marcia.

The one thing that the hospital tried to do—and that I completely understood—was to ensure that patients didn't stay in the emergency room for long because they needed those rooms for emergencies. They didn't even like having Marcia stay there that first night, and they kept looking for an available bed in the special care unit. Despite showing signs of improvement, it looked like Marcia would end up staying a second night in the emergency room due to a lack of space elsewhere. Late in the afternoon, they found a room in the special care unit for her.

We arrived in the new room late in the afternoon. Since Marcia had been on fluids for over a day, she had to use the bathroom as soon as we arrived. The nurse helped her to the bathroom and then came back into the room to get the bed ready. A minute or two later, the nurse and I heard a thud from the bathroom. We both hurried in and found that Marcia had fallen off the toilet. From that point on, I made sure that a nurse or I would be in the bathroom with Marcia.

YOU MUST HAVE AN ADVOCATE

The potty proved to be a bit of a struggle for me, and the potty won. I was emotionally hurt after I fell from the stool. The nurse should have been there watching me. She wasn't. Instead, she hurried to get my bed ready. After I fell, she quickly came into the bathroom to check to see that I was unscathed. Too late.

I've thought about this event a great deal and have concluded that she did the best she could. Perhaps she was stressed because they didn't have enough people on the floor that day. Or maybe it happened for some other reason. Regardless, it was clear to Jim and me that each patient in the hospital needs to have an advocate. For one thing, too much information is discussed during talks with providers. I wasn't able to remember much. Having an advocate to monitor those discussions took the pressure off me. Plus, having Jim's physical presence meant he could watch out for me and ensure I was never put in a dangerous situation. He never left my side, except when he went home to sleep.

JIM'S PERSPECTIVE

Marcia had the opportunity to order dinner the first night in her new room. The menu was very limited. I asked why. The stroke affected her throat and disabled the "sensor" that would make her cough if she started to choke. This meant she could easily choke on solid food, and without the warning cough, we'd never know. She could choke to death silently. Because of this, Marcia was only allowed to drink thick fluids or pureed food. With that simple explanation, the impact of Marcia's condition and her tenuous circumstances became clear. The fear finally hit me.

Up to sixty-five percent of stroke victims fail to swallow correctly (dysphagia) according to Thick'It. When these people swallow the food or drink might not move down the esophagus but may travel to the lungs by accident. Silent choking can occur, which can lead to dehydration, malnourishment, and pneumonia.[7]

DYSPHAGIA, OR CHOKING ON DINNER

In the ER, I was on intravenous fluids. By the time they transferred me to the special care unit, I'd graduated to "liquid food." (If you could call it food.) I had to sit upright and move my head to the left when I swallowed because of my weak neck muscles on the right side. I also had to take small drinks and clear my palate before I could take the next drink. I had to repeat this process each time. Jim watched me like a hawk. He didn't tell me why, though, and I didn't think to ask him. Obviously, he and the hospital staff worried that I'd choke.

Then, unexpectedly, I was given a real lunch. There was a mix up in the kitchen, and I received a tray of food. That meant I had to chew. Not surprisingly, I did choke briefly. The nursing staff didn't know I'd been given real food. When they discovered the mistake, they *chastised* me. How was I supposed to know that eating real food was a problem? My higher thinking skills had left the building. I was switched back to liquids. I'd say that I didn't notice much, but that would be a lie. It felt good having food that I could chew. I'd lost most of my taste buds, but I could smell the food. Besides, I could taste it enough to matter.

A NOTE FROM MARCIA

Approximately forty-eight people in the U.S. get dysphagia from stroke every single hour.

JIM'S PERSPECTIVE

When I left that evening, I called Marcia's sister, Dale. The night before, she hadn't known when she'd be able to travel to see Marcia. At that time, the earliest she could promise was the following weekend. After talking with her the second night, I asked if she could come sooner and she agreed. I'll always remember what I told her that night. "I was in the Air Force for twenty years. During those years, I had times when I was nervous, anxious, apprehensive, and other similar feelings, but never fear. Until tonight, I was never afraid."

I was afraid I'd, literally, have to stand by and watch Marcia die from doing something as simple as eating. The fear stayed with me for many weeks, to where I'd watch every bite she took to make sure she didn't choke to death. Later, when her cough "sensor" worked once again, and she'd choke and cough while eating, I didn't consider it a good sign. It just made me watch her even closer and repeatedly ask if she was okay.

CRYING BECAME MY NEW WAY OF LIFE

The physical changes were obvious. It soon became clear that something significant had changed for me emotionally. I cried a lot. Seriously, some things I cried over made no sense. I still often cry. Maybe that's a good thing because I'm now less shut off from the rest of the world.

ResearchGate reported that unchecked weeping is a natural aftereffect following a stroke. Practically anything emotional can prompt these crying jags, including seeing a loved one, seeing the doctor, sorrow, etc. Sometimes one cries for seemingly no reason.[8]

HOW ARE YOU AT READING, WRITING, AND SPEAKING?

The doctors and nurses visited my hospital room seemingly all the time armed with questions. "Can you raise your right hand? Good." "Can you write? It's interesting that you chose to write with your left hand." "Can you count? That's unusual. You're counting in Norwegian. You know, it would be better if you counted in your own language. Can you try that instead?"

I could write fairly well with my left hand. I had dislocated my right elbow in high school and had learned to write with my left hand to keep up with my schoolwork. I was able to count, too, but the hospital staff disliked that I chose to speak in Norwegian, the language I'd learned in college. Jim, on the other hand, was thrilled at the prospect of getting me back. He said this was when he knew I'd get better.

During one of these visits, someone commented that if I moved my right arm, the muscle wouldn't atrophy. Up. Down. Up. Down. I swung my right hand up above my head and back down to the bed somewhat rhythmically. The pain ignited in me, but I decided that I wouldn't let it stop me. I didn't want atrophy gumming up my style.

It wasn't until much later that I learned I'd be in constant pain for years. I had regular appointments with a massage therapist because I wanted my muscles to start working together in harmony. It was torture to lay on that table month after month after month. To the casual observer, I look like I walk normally, but things are still a little out of place. There's still pain in my hip, knee, and foot that I've learned to ignore. The moral of my story is that you shouldn't assume you know whether a stroke survivor feels pain or not based on how they look. Some stroke survivors have pain, some don't.

As I began my arm exercises in earnest, I knew I'd be healthy again. I had my family and friends, and I knew there was a higher purpose that had kept me on earth. I knew that I was going to write about my experience and that my story would help others.

The hospital staff also tried to get me to talk. At first, the words wouldn't come at all. I knew what I wanted to say. Sometimes I spoke short sentences and they came out just fine. Sometimes the words came out as gibberish. Sometimes I could think them, but saying the words escaped me. I'd sit silent, tired, and frustrated. At times, I felt incompetent. And the "trying" was exhausting. Many times, Jim had

to say the right words for me. I just didn't have the means to communicate well—but there was a good reason. I'd learn later that I had
aphasia and apraxia of speech.

"Aphasia is a disorder that results from damage to por-
tions of the brain that are responsible for language. For
most people, these areas are on the left side of the brain.
Aphasia usually occurs suddenly, often following a stroke
or head injury, but it may also develop slowly, as the result
of a brain tumor or a progressive neurological disease.
The disorder impairs the expression and understanding
of language as well as reading and writing. Aphasia may
co-occur with speech disorders, such as dysarthria or
apraxia of speech, which also result from brain damage."[9]

"Apraxia of speech (AOS)—also known as acquired
apraxia of speech, verbal apraxia, or childhood apraxia of
speech (CAS) when diagnosed in children—is a speech
sound disorder. Someone with AOS has trouble saying
what he or she wants to say correctly and consistently.
AOS is a neurological disorder that affects the brain pathways involved in planning the sequence of movements
involved in producing speech. The brain knows what it
wants to say but cannot properly plan and sequence the
required speech sound movements."[10]

JIM'S PERSPECTIVE

Several specialists helped put Marcia back on the road to recovery.
On many of these visits, the specialist would comment on how well
Marcia had improved. I was elated. When Marcia began speaking

Norwegian fluently, I saw that as a good sign for her recovery, even though the therapist required the responses in English.

A Note from Marcia

When you can think of the words clearly in your mind but you can't get them to come out of your mouth, you feel incompetent. There's nothing you can do. The more frustrated you become, the more likely you'll say nothing.

Jim's Perspective

Marcia would be in her hospital room for the next two and a half days, during which four noteworthy things happened.

First, I had to change my routines. To be honest, it wasn't that big of a deal. I had to become the caregiver. That meant taking care of the pets, paying bills, and ensuring all the plans for our future life were put in place. I established a new routine focused around Marcia and nothing else. I grabbed breakfast at Starbucks, which I ate in the hospital parking lot, and then spent the day with her, all of which I found enjoyable. The biggest gift came from the fact that I could be with Marcia.

Second, we realized how many close and dear friends we'd made in the area. We'd lived in the Metropolitan D.C. area for about twenty years and established a good group of friends, many from the various jobs that Marcia had held over the years. During Marcia's time in the special care ward, our friends knew they couldn't visit with her. However, a few select friends came to the hospital to make sure that I was doing all right. These visits came to mean a great deal to me and sealed the idea that these weren't only Marcia's good friends, but mine as well. They were friends whom I now think of as family.

A Note from Marcia

Friends are so important to the caregiver who's experiencing a whirlwind of emotions and may have trouble expressing feelings. The friends who visited Jim in the hospital gave him comfort, and we're both grateful for their kind words and actions.

Third, various specialists came to check on and work with Marcia. At least once each day, a neurologist or neural specialist talked with Marcia, since her stroke was so unexpected given her good health. Her stroke, a carotid artery dissection, had no known cause. It truly was spontaneous.

According to the Johns Hopkins Medicine website, those who experience arterial dissection have an aberrant, and frequently atypical, rupture along the inside wall of an artery. This rupture makes a tiny pocket called a "false lumen." Blood gathers within this false lumen and coagulates the blood, creating blood clots or obstruct blood flow, and eventually cause a stroke.[11]

Fourth, the hospital administrator immediately began working on finding a local rehabilitation hospital to which Marcia could be transferred. Although the main reason for their quick action on this was to free up the room, they also knew that getting a stroke victim into rehabilitation as quickly as possible is best for the patient. I worked with the administrator as she searched for a place for Marcia in the area. The only available hospital was quite a distance from our house, but we'd make it work.

WORKING MY RIGHT SIDE

On Tuesday, April 1, a physical therapist came to take me on another hospital walk. She put a belt around my waist, and we walked up and down the corridor. The klutz in me came out again. One foot in front of the other is harder than you think. So many muscles, tendons, and ligaments must fire correctly to get a smooth and steady gait.

My brain injury had completely muddled my ability to do anything synchronized on the right side of my body, and my gait was far from steady. I'd lost control of my right foot. Each time I took a step forward, the toes pointed down and slightly to the right. Once the step was taken, my foot drifted farther to the right while my left foot pointed straight ahead. My right knee hurt moderately, although it wasn't holding my attention. I felt an agonizing grinding of my right hip as I put my weight on it. My hip ground in a way that felt like bone on bone, as if someone had put an electric sander inside of me. Each movement was torture, and if I didn't understand what zero to ten meant on the pain scale before, I did now.

A Note from Marcia

As children, we learn to crawl and then walk. It's a process that we try, fail, try, fail, and try again. After a brain injury, you fail again and again and again as you relearn how the body works. Walking takes time and patience as muscles, tendons, and ligaments try to respond. Progress can be affected by tight and atrophied muscles on the affected side.

Cards, Flowers, Stuffed Animals, and Love

Jim kept the communication channels open with my friends and family. Each night, he'd communicate with my close friend, Donna Hemmert, whom I've worked with since our early days in Virginia. She kept that line of friends updated. He also texted Rochele, who communicated with my friends from George Mason University. Finally, he continued to have phone conversations with my sister. Just two days after my stroke, the flowers, cards, and stuffed animals began appearing in my room. The outpouring of love made me feel important.

For once, I knew how much my life meant to the people around me. I was humbled. It took time and effort to send each card and gift to me. The friends in my life loved me for who I was. I'll never forget that moment when I realized I wasn't really by myself. I had Jim. I had my family. I had my friends. Together, they would make living life sweet again.

Jim's Perspective

On Thursday morning, the hospital administrator said a room had opened at Bull Run Memorial, a new rehabilitation facility closer to our home. We needed to tell Bull Run Memorial if we planned to take the room, but Marcia had one more job to do first. She had to produce a stool sample. If she couldn't, she wouldn't be allowed to leave Greensboro Hospital. Being the trooper she is, and given that she hadn't produced one for five days, Marcia stepped up, or, more precisely, sat down and produced one successfully.

On to Bull Run Memorial

I hadn't bathed since Saturday morning, so the nurses made sure I took a "shower." They got some wet wipes and cleaned me up, kind of. They rubbed something in my hair and said I was ready to go. The hair thing was not spectacular. I was sporting a new style that no one would try. I didn't care, though. I was out of there!

It felt so freeing to get out of the hospital gown. Jim brought a set of workout clothes from home. They had a nice, tight fit, but that kind of clothing is a struggle to get in without having had a stroke! The nurse wrestled with both my top and bottom as I attempted to put them on. The final touches were my peridot green jacket and my purple sneakers. I was ready to roll! I just needed to wait for Jim to get everything packed in the car.

It took a couple of trips for Jim to put all the cards, plants, and stuffed animals into the car. Finally, the nurse wheeled me out of the room and out of the hospital. Although I struggled to get into the car, I was free. The air was refreshing, the antiseptic smell of the hospital vanishing from my nostrils as we drove away with the top down on the convertible. The day was bright and the sun shone warmly on my face. I looked around and marveled at the green grass and trees. Jim drove gently with me in the Solara, the wind tousling my hair. On Route 50, it got pretty rugged as miles of construction marred our drive to Bull Run Memorial. I was so joyous, I didn't care. Finally, Jim and I arrived.

JIM'S PERSPECTIVE

After gathering up the items that had accumulated in the room, we set off to the place for Marcia's next stage of rehabilitation. En route to the new rehab hospital, I was so happy to have Marcia in the car next to me and able to communicate, something that would have seemed unlikely just four days earlier.

TAKE ACTION

These steps are for you and the advocate/caregiver in your life. Each point is important and crucial to moving into this new reality with grace and patience.

- Keep a set of medical records on hand. Your advocate will need to know your medical history, the medicines and supplements you take, the allergies you have, etc.

- Talk about a healthcare directive with someone who is qualified if you want to have control over how your care is managed, and under what circumstances you'd like to refuse further care. We didn't have this important document, which also would have contained a "Do Not Resuscitate," also called a "DNR," requirement in the event things went sideways. DNR rules vary by state. Please consult an attorney.

- Know what your insurance covers. Not everyone is as lucky as we were.

- Have an advocate. You'll be working hard to heal. You may not hear things properly or be able to respond clearly. An advocate will not only listen and talk for you but will also be there to make sure you're protected from physical calamity.

- Accept help from friends and family. They can be a supreme source of support for you and the caregiver.

- Appreciate the people in your life.

- Establish a short list of people who can communicate with others. Having these intermediary contacts will allow your caregiver to spend most of their time with you and not talking on the phone.

- Sleep as much as possible when you are taking care of someone else. It might seem odd, but caregivers need to rest so that they can continue being a strong advocate.

- Get time off from work. Caregiving can be hard, especially when it comes to asking for time off. Having a caregiver by your side every day will make a huge difference.

- Ask questions if you're a caregiver and the instructions aren't clear. Medical terminology can be confusing, especially to a non-medical person. Always ask what a doctor, nurse, or specialist means. It's okay to ask them to put their words into laymen's terms.

- Stay calm in the hospital room. Caregivers are meant to be supportive.

- Have patience. Stroke affects every person differently. It can even change a person's personality. Communicating can be hard. Caregivers should listen, watch, and be there for the patient.

- Responsibilities and household adjustments happen. Caregiving doesn't end when the patient leaves the hospital. Often, changes at home regarding roles and responsibilities must happen. Some may be temporary; others permanent.

Chapter 3

MOVING ON TO REHABILITATION

Jim parked at the door when we got to Bull Run Memorial. He went in while I waited. It didn't take long for the nursing staff to come with a wheelchair for me. I carefully maneuvered my way out of the car and into the wheelchair. Impressed, the nurse complimented my ability to move.

I noticed the unmistakable antiseptic "hospital" smell as she wheeled me to my room. I had a nice corner room with a single bed and sunshine streaming through the window. I sat patiently in the wheelchair as the hospital staff told us what to expect. They put my stats on two whiteboards. One board had all the people I'd be working with and what they did. The therapists would keep track of my progress day by day. The other had the doctor on duty, the nurse on duty, the person who I would call if I needed assistance, and my goals to get better.

I was told I'd be in there for a week. If my therapists thought I needed more therapy, they'd ask for another week. I'd be doing physical therapy, occupational therapy, and speech therapy. I also would eat in the dining room, and Jim could eat there, too. The first night, though, I ate liquid food in the room, and Jim ate hospital food.

It helped that my nurse from Greensboro Hospital had a connection with my nurse at Bull Run Memorial. Even better, both had a linkage to someone at our insurance agency. Their connections made it much easier to transition out of Greensboro and into Bull Run Memorial.

Jim's Perspective

I immediately liked Bull Run Memorial. The newness and cleanliness of the facility made me happy. Then, once Marcia had settled into her room, the structure of the facility's operations impressed me. One of the first things they did was introduce the various staff members, including the resident physician Marcia would be interacting and working with daily. These introductions allowed Marcia (and me) to recognize the faces of her nurses and therapists and match the names on her whiteboard with those faces.

That first night, I'm sure Marcia had some trepidation about what would be happening during her stay at the rehab hospital, but she didn't show it much. Whether her lack of emotion was an effect from the stroke or just her approach to life, I'll probably never know. I do know that I didn't want to leave her there alone that first night, and I felt an emptiness in my stomach as I left.

Getting Started

Jim arrived with more clothes on Friday morning. I've always been terribly afraid of disrobing in front of people I don't know. Now, I didn't have a choice. I realized that I didn't care as much as I thought I would. The occupational therapist (OT) wheeled me into my bathroom, disrobed me, turned the water on, and helped me from my chair to the seat in the shower. She handed me the soap and said, "Take as much time as you need." Then she closed the curtain and waited patiently.

Ah! That hot water feels so nice running down my back! I thought. I spent a long time soaking in the steaming water. It had been nearly a week since my last shower. I absolutely needed to feel the warmth hitting my skin and rinsing the sweat off my body. Moving the bar of soap around was comical as it almost slipped out of my hand several times. I did my best, but the soap didn't get everywhere it should have. My feet and back simply got the runoff. Despite not being entirely clean, it still felt like heaven!

A NOTE FROM MARCIA

When it came right down to the truth, I didn't care much about personal privacy anymore because it was a luxury. This type of luxury was no longer possible.

The next thing I had to do was wash my hair, which still had that awful goop in it that the Greensboro nurse had used the day before. I couldn't wait to get it out! Washing my hair took a long time because I couldn't use my right hand to reach my scalp. I used the shampoo dispenser and got my left hand ready. I shampooed twice and then rinsed out the suds. When I finished, I called the OT. After the shower, I felt clean—amazing, really—and I didn't smell bad anymore.

The OT dried me off and rolled me into my room. That's when we realized that Jim had only brought workout clothes. The jog bra was a pain to get on because it rolled over onto itself. It took a long time for the OT to unroll it and put it into place. The shirt was a bit odd as well because it stretched. I did like how the yoga pants fit, however.

Finally dressed, it was time for the morning ablutions. It was dreadful. That's the only word that describes combing my hair. It was grown out, stringy, and snarled. I hadn't been given any conditioner to tame my hair, which meant I could barely get the comb through it.

Next came tooth brushing. My teeth needed a good cleaning. I put the toothpaste on the brush. It didn't dump all over the sink. I started brushing with my right hand, but it had a mind of its own. It wasn't long before I switched to the left hand, but I made a mess with that one, too. The worst part was when I tried to get the toothpaste out of my mouth, I kept spitting on my hand. Even though I told my right hand to move, it took longer for me to move it out of the way than it did for my spit to drop. It took me quite a while to learn that spitting in the sink and arm movement had to be coordinated. When I finished, I had to use a washcloth to clean my mouth, my right arm, and my hand. I'm pretty sure my teeth didn't get brushed all that well, either, but I was proud that I'd accomplished this task by myself.

Going to the bathroom presented new opportunities to relinquish my privacy. Just as the nurses in Greensboro had helped me, the nurses at Bull Run Memorial also ensured my safety, unless Jim was there. When he wasn't, I had to ring the nursing staff. They made sure I rolled my way into the bathroom. They helped me get out of my wheelchair, steadied me as I turned around, took my pants down, and made sure I was sitting on the stool safely. They left me alone while I did my business. In the beginning, even using toilet paper was hard. Trying to roll the toilet paper and wipe was almost beyond me. After doing my business, I'd need assistance again. I'd ring the bell, and they'd come back to help get me in the wheelchair again.

The mattress at Bull Run Memorial was covered with a plastic sheet for those who had incontinent issues. (There are some things to be thankful for, and I didn't have that particular problem.) Getting comfortable was a challenge, though. Comfort no longer existed for me. I was in agony because the pain in my right side was always present. The trick was finding postures that made me less miserable.

A Note from Marcia

The stroke changed the way I perceived pain. My right side was affected; it moved with short, choppy motions from my right foot to my facial muscles. Over time, the movements became smoother, and it became less obvious I'd had a stroke.

My right side wasn't universally affected. The most to least affected areas were the shoulder, hip, wrist, knee, foot. The more afflicted a body part was the more attention it got. I focused on my shoulder. After a long time, my focus moved to my hip, and so on. As my movements became more fluid, people thought the pain had also gone away. It hadn't. The pain is always there. It's diminished, but it's taken years. I don't notice it much now because there are so many more important things to do and feel.

When I needed to go to the bathroom or simply wanted to get out of bed, I'd use the call button. The nurse would come in and watch me as I inched my way across the bed. I'd move a few inches with my left side. Then I'd have to work to get my right leg to catch up. Then I'd repeat the process. When I finally made it to the edge of the bed, I had to figure out how to get into the wheelchair. Dragging myself across the bed to get in or out was an ordeal, but I got the hang of it as the days passed.

When I got up in the morning, the nurse would make my bed and put the stuffed animals on top. In a way, I think that process helped me stay out of bed for most days because I didn't want to mess it up.

The control panel for the bed also allowed me to work the TV. At first, only Jim would use the TV while I was out of the room for therapy. Eventually, I turned it on at night for the noise. I wasn't interested in what was showing, though. A rehab hospital is a lonely place at night, and the noise made me feel less deserted.

My Therapies

Being in a rehabilitative hospital meant it was time for me to get to work on regaining what I'd lost. I had speech, physical, and occupational therapy every day.

I went to speech therapy after showering on the first day. Mandy, the speech therapist, stepped into my room, introduced herself, and wheeled me down to her office. She took her time getting to know me. Although I didn't speak much, I clearly knew most of the answers to the questions she asked. We talked about apraxia and aphasia. She told me that I had both. I'm part of approximately forty percent of stroke survivors who have a communication disorder. Mine impairs my ability to process language.

A Note from Marcia

Nearly 30 people per hour get some kind of speech impediment caused by stroke in the United States.

We proceeded to go through some exercises, so she could get a sense of what I knew. Where I had the most trouble was getting things to roll off my tongue. She gave me exercises to do with Jim, such as how to count. I spoke the big words better than the little words. "S" words threw me off, as did "N" words because they were difficult to say. It was challenging, but it was also fun. Although speech therapy only lasted an hour, I was pooped when she rolled me back to my room where Jim was waiting patiently to see me.

Physical therapy was done in a large room, and I shared my therapist with another person. The physical therapist put a belt on me and we walked around the room. Sometimes she'd put me on a hand cycle to pedal for ten minutes. All the therapies were hard, but I felt pretty good when I finished. As I got stronger, she'd challenge me more.

Instead of walking around the room with me, we'd walk up and down a set of steps located in the center of the room.

While physical therapy was designed to help me carry out big and small movements to reteach my body how to be coordinated, occupational therapy helped me relearn those everyday tasks—those things we do almost automatically because they're so ingrained. Occupational therapy was the hardest for me. I had to relearn how to do things like going to the bathroom, tying my shoes, and taking a shower. I had to clip and unclip things, and I had to get things into bowls without using my right hand. I stunk at occupational therapy, but the OT kept encouraging me. Over time, I did see improvement.

FAMILY TIME

Jim always held his emotions in check when he was with me. In the early days, he left his anxiety at the door—as much as he could. In time, I noticed that he choked up when he talked to people, including my sister. During their nightly text, she asked if she and my brother-in-law needed to come to visit me. The answer was yes. It wasn't the best time of year for a CPA to leave her practice, but she and Joel were coming anyway.

DALE'S PERSPECTIVE

When Jim finally called, it was good news. Marcia's speech was garbled, but she could talk. She was also able to move her arms and legs, and she was cognizant. He called again later that evening with an update. I immediately called Keith so that he could pass the information on to the rest of his family. We were all so relieved, but we knew she wasn't out of the woods yet.

By Monday evening, she seemed to have improved a little more. There were still so many things that could go wrong to cause her to take a turn for the worst. We were all scared. I continued to update Keith and his family. Jim and I started texting.

Joel and I decided we were both going to visit, in part because Joel would've been worried and anxious at home. Although Marcia needed her family by her side, Jim needed us just as much, even if it was for only a few days. Marcia's stroke was traumatic for him, too, and he needed family support, not just support from the medical professionals. Besides, with Joel there, we'd have a foursome to play cards.

Jim and I discussed who needed to know the news of Marcia's stroke. He agreed it was important that our aunt and cousins were told. Both of our parents came from small families, each having only one sibling. Our parents were both gone, but Dad's sister, Esther, was still living. At age ninety-six, she could still beat all of us at cards. Dad and Esther had been close and used to talk to each other every day. I knew she'd want to know about Marcia's stroke. On Tuesday morning, I called her oldest daughter, Bev, and used her as the information conduit. She relayed the news to her mom and her sister. I promised that I'd keep them updated even if there wasn't a lot of news. Sometimes, just knowing things haven't worsened is a comfort.

We were delighted to hear that Marcia would be moving to a rehab center on Thursday. She'd been approved for a week of extensive rehab. Only five days had passed since her stroke on Sunday to her discharge to rehab. Marcia's life had changed in ways we couldn't imagine. She'd been self-employed with a growing business before Sunday. Now her job would be to regain what the stroke had taken from her.

Our paternal grandmother was seventy-seven when she had a stroke so serious that she died almost instantly. She never got the chance for rehab. We also had a great uncle who had a stroke at approximately the same age. He made it to rehab. I remember visiting Harold after his stroke. He had difficulty speaking, eating, and walking, and died later that summer. Marcia was only fifty-three but hadn't suffered Grandma's fate. I hoped she wouldn't suffer Harold's fate either. I wanted her to work hard to recover all the skills she'd lost so that she could enjoy life again. Perhaps her younger age and physical fitness would allow for this to happen.

On Friday morning, we began our cross-country flight. Jim met us at the gate and we headed for the rehab hospital, stopping only for a fast food supper. Jim warned us that Marcia looked different and to not be surprised. When I saw her, I thought she looked super. Her smile was a little lopsided, but it was there. She looked just like herself, and we were so happy to see her. True, her speech had been affected, and she also had some difficulty with strength and coordination on her right side. But she was sitting up and talking to us.

Her rehab had already begun, and she had three rehab therapy sessions a day. Joel and I brought our own brand of therapy. Esther introduced us to a rummy game, so in her honor, it's called "Esther's rummy." It's a real brain workout as the hands dealt get progressively bigger: three cards are dealt, then four, then five, up to thirteen. Then there are the rules. With three cards, the threes are wild; with four cards, the fours are wild, etc. When thirteen cards are dealt, the kings are wild. By playing cards, we helped Marcia work on both her speech and physical therapy. We also made her count points for all of us, and she had to hold her cards, which isn't easy for even the non-stroke survivor when the hands consist of twelve or thirteen cards. When she made a mistake, we'd help her count correctly. We also added a twist to the game. When a wild card was thrown away by mistake, the person would receive a half "stupid" point. We waived this rule for Marcia, and when she threw a wild card, we pointed it out and let her have the card back. I was happy that she won many games that weekend.

The rehab hospital allowed visitors from 9:00 a.m. to 9:00 p.m. We were there for only the weekend so we spent all the time we could at the rehab, leaving only when they took Marcia for meals. Joel and I brought her a stuffed giraffe. Its legs were weighted so it could stand. Like the giraffe had to stretch to reach tasty leaves in the trees, Marcia would need to stretch her abilities to regain what she had lost. It was so good to see her, and it was difficult to watch her struggle to find the words she wanted. Even in just two days, I could see that she was improving. I want to think that our visit aided in her recovery.

Jim told us that it was good for him to have us there. After spending the day with Marcia, we'd go to Jim and Marcia's house where we'd spend time talking with him and enjoying a little wine. Marcia wasn't the only one needing us. Jim was scared. No one knew what Marcia's long-term prognosis would be, and her stroke would have a major impact on Jim's life as well. He'd need to be a caregiver for at least the short-term. This would be a different role for him, but one he was glad to assume, knowing that playing this role was better than what the alternative could have been.

These late evening conversations helped each of us. One thing I could do was to file their income tax extension, as Marcia was the one who did their taxes. Because she had her stroke at the end of March, she already had most of the information together. I pulled it all together and filed the extension. We could cross that off of Jim's worry list.

We flew home on Monday. Jim reported that after we left, Marcia was able to walk with a cane during physical therapy. That week, she also graduated to being able to eat in her room, instead of being watched like a hawk in the dining room to ensure she didn't choke.

Marcia also started sending me texts the week after I left. The aphasia had affected her written speech, too. Sometimes the words or syntax she used was incorrect, but that was immaterial. She was able to type on her itty-bitty phone! When I got a text from her, it meant she was okay. I didn't have to worry that she'd had a big setback. That knowledge was important to me.

My text to Marcia:

> *We just got home. It was good to see you and Jim. We're so pleased to see the progress you're making.*
>
> *Love,*
> *Dale*

Marcia's text to me:

> *We good few lunch learn.*

When I got home, I called Esther to let her know that Marcia was still able to win at "Esther's rummy." She was happy to get a personal update from me about Marcia.

A Note from Marcia

I was so proud when I texted Dale, although sometimes the texts didn't make sense. The most difficult thing I had to do when preparing my daily dialogue was remembering the password on my phone. Sometimes I would remember it, no problem. Sometimes I couldn't think of it for hours. It was so frustrating! Not remembering happens when you have a brain injury.

Jim's Perspective

Monday marked the last day of the visit from Dale and Joel, as well as the last day I'd be able to spend all day with Marcia. As she settled into her new rehabilitation routine, I began a new routine at work. For the next eight workdays, as I had been on a work schedule of ten-hour days for four days a week, I worked six hours and took leave for the remaining four hours. I was out of the office by noon every day. I grabbed some food to eat in the car and arrived at the hospital around 1:30 p.m. I was glad to see Marcia and curious to see how she'd progressed.

Because I was with Marcia during work hours, I was able to see some of the therapists working with her and watch her progress in her recovery. It gave me great comfort knowing that Marcia was in good hands in my absence. As the second week rolled around, they let me assist Marcia in completing some of the physical therapy. The knowledge I gained would come in handy for the next stage of Marcia's rehabilitation.

The optimum next stage of rehabilitation was to begin outpatient therapies at a qualified location. However, finding a location, even with some help from the rehabilitation hospital staff, proved difficult. Our best option was to get on a waiting list, which gave no guarantees of getting a slot. So, we scheduled some therapists to work with Marcia in-home, until we could get her into an outpatient slot somewhere.

A Note from Marcia

I had to take baby aspirin (an antiplatelet drug, which means it prevents blood from clotting as easily), Metoprolol succinate (a beta-blocker that affects the heart and circulation), and a statin (reduces cholesterol) when I was in the hospital and rehab hospital. I didn't have high cholesterol, so I talked to my doctor about the statin after I left the rehab hospital. We agreed to stop that medication. You have a right to question treatments, scans, drugs, tests, and understand what they're trying to alleviate. If you don't agree with the answer, you have a right to get a second opinion.

REHAB ROUTINE

My days were packed: breakfast, medicine, shower. Then, the ablutions aka trying not to spit on my hand. After that, comb my hair—or try to. Then off to therapy, lunch in the cafeteria, and then more therapy. Finally, time off with Jim, dinner in the cafeteria, and then rummy with Jim until he left at 7:00 or 8:00 p.m. I received another round of medicine and was totally ready for bed.

While it doesn't seem like much to do for a day, it was tough. All I wanted to do was sleep sometimes. Although the therapy time was truncated by having to share the PT and OT with other patients, I was completely exhausted when I finished. But I loved speech therapy! It didn't matter how well (or poorly) I did each day, I always wanted to do more.

The therapists were great, too. It mattered that they deeply cared about my well-being. I was generally in a good mood. I'd been in Bull Run Memorial for about a week, and, as my time wound down, it was clear that I'd need one more week so that I could continue making substantial progress. As promised, Bull Run Memorial took care of it—no muss or fuss from our end.

By this time, I was eating pureed foods like oatmeal, scrambled eggs, and mashed potatoes, which meant I needed to manage a utensil. Breakfast came, and the staff would crank up my bed. I'll be honest; I usually ate with my left hand. Having lived in Norway for ten months in college, switching the fork side came naturally to me. I tried to eat with my right hand, too, but most of the time, the food fell off my fork. Before the stroke, I would've said that I wanted to drop fifteen pounds. I don't recommend having a stroke as a weight loss solution!

As I improved physically, the PTs made me do more challenging activities. I had to pull rings over a flexible bar using my right hand and bring them back again. I had to go up and down the stairs. Jim told me that I forgot to use my cane sometimes. Oops! As long as I didn't hit anyone, I guess it was probably okay.

JIM'S PERSPECTIVE

To ensure that Marcia was in a safe environment at home, two of the therapists came to our house the day before her release to evaluate its safety and to determine whether the safety features added were enough. For the most part, I only had to make minor modifications. I needed to buy a cane and put a seat in the shower. The next day, I brought Marcia, her menagerie of stuffed animals, and her greenhouse of plants and flowers home. Finally.

HOME

I left Bull Run Memorial on a balmy day. I couldn't wait to get home. With the convertible top down, the blowing breeze felt so good on my face. I couldn't believe the trees had leaves! As we drove, I realized once again how lucky I was to have Jim taking care of me.

When we got to the house, we waited in the car for the occupational and physical therapists to arrive. When they got there, they watched as I muddled my way out of the car. The seatbelt dug across my middle. The door was heavy and I had to swing it open with my left hand. Getting out was much harder than getting in. Looking back, I said I was at sixty percent. I realized that was a lie. I kept telling myself that, and I believe that lie carried me forward.

We walked through the garage toward the door into the house. Everyone looked at the step with no railing. "This could be a problem," the physical therapist said. "Careful. Always go out with your right foot first, and make sure you have your cane." I looked at our one step with no railing apprehensively. I took my time. Eventually, I made it through the door.

"Oh, look! You have a cat!" the OT said. Pharaoh yowled when he saw me. "Where have you been? Why have you been gone so long? Pet me! I said, Pet Me!" Pharaoh had been my companion for seventeen years. Now, old and frail, he didn't understand why I'd been gone so long. He let me know he didn't like this imposition.

We walked upstairs after I finished petting Pharaoh. We live in a split-level house, which means you must go up or down steps to get anywhere. "Take your time. Use your cane. You did okay on that, but Jim had better watch you for a while, especially with the cat hovering between your feet," both therapists cautioned me.

We made our way to the bedroom and adjacent bathroom. A new chair stood at the back of the shower. As the therapists and Jim looked at the shower and had their discussion, I held Pharaoh again. I had missed him so much! I also lay down on the bed. I learned, at that moment, that our waterbed would not work for me in my current condition. Lying down wasn't a problem but getting up was an ordeal. I rolled around for a while, trying to find some purchase. Jim finally had to help me get up.

JIM'S PERSPECTIVE

As time goes by, many of the events of those two and a half weeks become harder to remember. But it's fascinating how a few of those events remain crystal clear in my mind. It's amazing how a memory can stick with you so strongly when it's linked to an emotion.

By the time Marcia returned home, she could walk, talk, and do everyday tasks. The rehabilitation hospital and any subsequent therapies focused on just these three aspects of Marcia's recovery. Although doing so did allow her to get back to doing things on her own, there was no weight training to keep her muscles from atrophying.

Marcia immediately started in-home rehabilitation. She met with therapists for six weeks. I have to admit, and subsequently have had others agree with me, that some of the in-home therapies weren't that useful. The PT and OT therapists who worked with Marcia to improve her ambulatory abilities and dexterity didn't really offer anything that Marcia couldn't have done on her own. However, working with them was better than nothing. The exception was speech therapy. We were very pleased with the speech therapist who helped Marcia get her speaking ability back. The changes were noticeable, which also boosted Marcia's confidence.

Two issues worth noting took place during her in-home therapy. First, while Marcia was using the in-home therapies, she was considered a homebound patient due to insurance regulations. This meant that she couldn't leave the house at all except for doctor appointments during that period.

Second, I kept searching for other outpatient therapy locations that worked with stroke patients. By chance, someone told me that one of the local hospitals did this type of therapy, yet that hospital wasn't on the list of locations given to me by the rehabilitation hospital. I jumped on the opportunity and inquired about availability. While Marcia would have to go without therapy for a week or two after the in-home completed, she was on this new location's schedule.

Would it Happen Again?

The neurologists will tell you they don't know why my carotid artery tore. My cholesterol levels were in the normal range. I used to have high blood pressure that was controlled by medication, but through exercise and meditation, my blood pressure had been in the normal range for quite a while. I'd been off the medication for months without a hitch. I guess the "why did this happen?" question will remain a mystery.

Jim worried about it. The stroke happened once. Would it happen again? A few weeks after I was released from Bull Run Memorial, I went to Prosperity Hospital to get a different neurologist's opinion. Jim looked relieved when the neurologist confirmed that the blood flow between the lower and upper left carotid artery had been severed and said that blood flow wouldn't return. This particular neurologist was wrong.

TAKE ACTION

- Accept help. When you're in early recovery, chances are that you need to let someone bathe you, help dress you, and possibly assist you when going to the bathroom. You may feel a bit uncomfortable, but those things need to be done. I understood how dependent I was on other people after my stroke. Being dependent also made me want to get better, so I wouldn't need their help. Freedom is a great motivator.

- Get out of the hospital gown. In my opinion, there's nothing as degrading as a hospital gown when you're sick. Getting dressed made me feel more alive. At this stage, every little thing helps.

- Clean yourself every single day. By now, you know that you can only do so much. Getting out of bed, showering, dressing, brushing your teeth, and combing your hair before you go back to bed may take you all day (with naps in between each step). That's fine. Just do it.

- Move around. Sometimes it's as simple as getting off your bed and into the wheelchair or using a cane or walker. Maybe you can't go very far, but you might go farther the next day. Over time, these little victories add up. You may not walk fast, but you'll put in a mile or two (or more) over time.

- Allow your emotions to show. Seeing family for the first time may bring out a whole host of emotions. Let them happen. You might feel vulnerable after your stroke. I know I did. I cried when my family came; I cried when they left. I wasn't unhappy to see them, but the only emotion I seemed to express clearly involved crying.

- Playing games is an excellent form of therapy. My family bent the rules for Esther's rummy and I occasionally won. Winning felt awesome!

- Try to remember your password. If your phone or tablet are like mine, they have a password. Short-term memory can be hard to come by after you've had a stroke. I know it was for me. Perhaps it might have helped to sing the password. I sat for a long time every day, trying to remember what it was. When I had it, I could text to my sister, which gave me great joy.

- Snuggle with your pet (if you have one). Your pet doesn't care that you're not all there. If I wanted to cry, my cat snuggled with me. He let me know I wasn't alone. If you don't have a pet, consider getting an older dog or cat.

- Sleep where you're the most comfortable. I know people probably found it odd that I slept on an air mattress on the living room floor. Sleeping in the waterbed was awkward for me. It was just too hard to get out of it.

- Admit mistakes. The neurologist I saw said the blood flow through my carotid artery wouldn't come back. But it did. You need to recognize that doctors only know what they know, and they're still learning, especially when it comes to the brain. You also need to realize that you, too, make mistakes.

- Be kind. Working in hospitals and rehab hospitals is challenging. If someone makes a mistake that's not life-threatening, let it go. You have other things to worry about on your road to recovery.

Chapter 4

LEARNING TO SPEAK

I don't know how other people feel after they've had a stroke, but I thought for sure I'd be back to my old self by the first anniversary. I tried my darnedest, but I wasn't my old self by the first anniversary, or the second, or the third. The problem was that I wanted to be the person I'd been before the stroke. It took quite a while before I finally admitted that she didn't exist anymore.

That said, everyone told me that the greatest progress I'd make in recovery would come during the first year. Bull Run Memorial started me on my journey with speech, occupational, and physical therapies. Now that I was home, Jim arranged for me to continue with home health providers who could take care of it all. This chapter chronicles how I progressed through speech therapy at Bull Run Memorial followed by home healthcare, and outpatient care at local hospitals. The next two chapters focus on occupational and physical therapies using the same structure, including finally paying for a physical therapist on my own because I thought I needed a lot more training to be mobile.

SPEECH THERAPY AT BULL RUN MEMORIAL (APRIL 4 TO APRIL 18, 2014)

I really liked my speech therapist at Bull Run Memorial. Confident, caring, and clever, Mandy worked me hard. I went from single words to very short sentences. When I had trouble with a word, she gave me space and time to work through my issue. Sometimes I couldn't think of any response. I remember lying to her about eggs—I just don't like them. I couldn't think of the exact words I wanted to say when she asked about breakfast. I'd been eating eggs every day in rehab, so they were on my mind. She also had me repeat sounds that I couldn't pronounce well, especially sounds at the end of a word like "ng" and "th."

According to Wikipedia, Word selection anomia happens when the stroke patient understands how an item operates, can choose the item from an arrangement of items, and still cannot label it correctly.[12]

Mandy gave me lots of puzzles to do with my husband. Jim would ask me questions like:

- Who flies planes?
- Who puts out fires?
- Who delivers mail?

Sometimes I could come up with a name. Sometimes I drew a blank. Jim would also ask questions designed to create lists of similar items. It wasn't as easy as it sounds. He'd ask about a variety of things.

- Articles of clothing? That I could do.
- Foods? You bet.

- Animals? Easy, because I had some stuffed animals on my bed.
- Sports? Not so much.

As I had experienced with Mandy, I sometimes got the words right, while sometimes I couldn't think of anything. I often got stuck with synonyms and antonyms. I just couldn't figure them out. Jim and I played cards when I needed a break.

I also had problems remembering things. I might have just spoken to someone and I couldn't remember what they'd said. It was really frustrating when I couldn't remember simple things like the passcode to my iPad and iPhone. One minute I had it; the next it was lost. I could remember having the passcode on the tip of my tongue, but then I'd forget it before I typed it. Sometimes it took hours before I remembered the login.

"Cognitive impairment and memory loss are common after a stroke. Approximately 30% of stroke patients develop dementia within 1 year of stroke onset. Stroke affects the cognitive domain, which includes attention, memory, language, and orientation. The most affected domains are attention and executive functions; at the time of stroke diagnosis, memory problems are often prominent."[13]

When Jim and I left Bull Run Memorial, Mandy included this note in my file:

At this time, patient requires minimum to moderate assist for verbal expression tasks, specifically sentence formulation and responding to complex "Wh" interrogatives: who, why, how, when, where, and what. Patient continues to demonstrate some perseveration of previously stated words/phrases; however, patient demonstrates marked improvement in the area. When speaking with unfamiliar people, patient's difficulty is maximized. Patient is discharged home tomorrow with her husband.

Safety considerations: Have someone assist you with daily finances. Have someone assist you with your medications.

Her comment about safety considerations was important. Not only had I experienced a stroke, but I was also dyslexic. Paying bills wouldn't have made sense to me. I don't even know if I could've written a check in April 2014. Because of my foggy memory, her comment about medications made perfect sense. I needed someone to remember when I took my meds. It required too much logical thinking to remember if, or when, I'd taken them.

Although the Speech Therapy Discharge Instructions read as if I was better, I think talking turned out to be my biggest challenge. After calling around to some of the places provided to us by Bull Run Memorial, Jim arranged for home care to start on Monday, April 21. During my short waiting period, I did some of the exercises on my own.

According to AskWonder, there's a distinction between Broca's and Wernicke's aphasia. Broca's aphasia deals with motor speech. Stroke survivors comprehend what's said by other people, but they can't generate sounds or language themselves. Wernicke's aphasia is sensory in nature. Stroke survivors with Wernicke's aphasia can create speech themselves, but they can't understand what others are saying.[14]

I don't know if it is so difficult for other people to understand the difference between apraxia and aphasia. Here is what I now understand: Apraxia has to do with speech, how the individual communicates sounds and words. It has to do with the way the lips, tongue, and mouth are shaped; the breath and vocal cords making sounds; and cadence. Aphasia deals with language processing, which brings other people into the equation.

SPEECH THERAPY AT HOME (APRIL 21 TO JUNE 5, 2014)

When I met Kim, I knew that she was someone I could trust. A recent Seattle transplant, she took her job seriously and made working together fun. She focused on my ability to say small words. Sometimes being overeducated gives you a disadvantage. I really liked to say the big words, but they often tripped me up.

Kim gave me books to read (and reread), often written by Dr. Seuss. She liked these books because they had unpronounceable words for a stroke patient. Try as I might, I often got stuck on these words.

As my speech improved, she upgraded the books so that I had to work harder. When we finished my therapy, I had been reading *Fox in Socks* for a couple of weeks and got it mostly right.

I also started learning words through rhymes.

- Peter Piper picked a peck of pickled peppers . . .
- Four furious friends fought for the phone.
- I scream, you scream, we all scream for ice cream! (Yeah, I liked this one!)

In addition to reading Dr. Seuss for speech therapy, Kim also encouraged me to read books on my own. I remember reading *Focus: The*

Hidden Driver of Excellence by Dan Goleman. I love his work! While I read quite well in silence, my brain messed up when I tried to read aloud. Even more frustrating was that I couldn't remember a single thing about what I'd read. I was confused as to how I could understand the written word but not remember it.

Kim also had me read documents I'd written before the stroke. Although I had dyslexia, my mother had me read aloud to her for years. So, my pre-stroke writing was edgy, clear, and elegant. Reading my blog posts, websites, and other materials, it seemed impossible that I could have written words so eloquently. And yet I did!

There was a real difference between reading the words (which I could do) and remembering how to write them. It seemed as if I could no longer spell. To get beyond that, Kim had me play games like Scrabble. Everybody had to play by the rules except me. I had all the time in the world to come up with a word. If I misspelled a word, other players would tell me, and I'd pick up my pieces and try again. Playing Scrabble with me made people wince. They participated anyway, and I'm grateful that they showed me so much compassion.

The exercises I worked on under Kim's care were harder than the ones at Bull Run Memorial. She told me to look at the use and function of the word. I needed to be obvious about what the words said. The "wh" words continued to give me some problems. I needed to think about location, what the object looked like, or who used it as I wrapped my brain around the words I needed to capture.

Kim gave me words that were more challenging to practice. These tested my patience and included words such as influenza, flotilla, and bumblebee. She also had me continue my word endings practice that I'd begun at Bull Run Memorial. I still had trouble pronouncing word endings, which had something to do with speaking loud enough. It took a long while before anyone could hear me when I spoke in public.

Kim also told me to look up words when I was stuck. I relearned how to use an online thesaurus site to aid in my practice. I got stuck a lot. Sometimes I couldn't even spell the word I knew, so using the thesaurus consumed many hours.

Exercises to explain what a person does with an item became part of my daily routine. I had to think through what a plunger did, how binoculars make a difference in how you see things, and where an eraser works.

Kim told me to take my time thinking of the words, just like Mandy had. She told me to slow down, and if I was stuck, that I should think about ways to say the same thing differently. In fact, she didn't think it was reasonable for me to expect to talk as fast as I used to.

Like everything else in speech therapy, all these exercises challenged me. It took a long time for me to say words correctly. I practiced my reading, writing, nursery rhymes, and games every day. By June 5, Kim said she'd given me the keys to "getting better." I'd need to continue practicing, but she honestly felt that I had what I needed for the road to recovery. It was a long road. Unfortunately, Kim misread my progress.

SPEECH THERAPY AT HOPE HOSPITAL (MAY 5 TO JUNE 24, 2015)

During my first anniversary checkup with my neurologist, my doctor decided that I needed additional therapy. I was frustrated because I couldn't get my words quite right. Although my checkup was in March, my therapy didn't start until May. It seemed like a long time to wait.

I was nervous when I approached Anita for the first time. I had the right to be apprehensive, after all, I'd been through speech therapy twice already. Although the therapy only lasted eight weeks, Anita tried her best to stump me. And stump me she did! Anita worked on the hardest words and phrases she had. Sometimes I drew a blank still. Taking my time to think of the words helped me. By the end of six weeks, I had a reason for standing up and speaking in public.

By this time, the interstate behind our home had become a point of contention for me. The state was planning to widen the highway, and that meant our backyard would be cut in half. The first planning meeting happened while I was working with Anita. I worked with her to express myself, succinctly, in public. On the day of the meeting, I signed up to speak. When they called my name, I stood up, grabbed my notes, and walked slowly toward the podium. I looked out at the crowd. My heart pounded. I had three minutes to explain how this construction would devastate our yard and our house. I had to slow down two or three times, but I spoke loudly enough to be heard. I stumbled on a word or two, but I didn't give up. It felt fantastic to get what I was feeling deep down off my chest.

The next time I had speech therapy, Anita lauded me for my accomplishment. She believed I'd learned enough from her. Little did she know that I still had a long, long way to go. Doing exercises isn't the same thing as speaking. Although I did the exercises well, what I thought and what I said were often two separate entities. When I was tired or felt annoyed, I couldn't project what I thought. I'd get angry and speak less. I would sometimes, literally, say nothing.

According to the Journal of Cognitive and Behavioral Neurology, we interpret sounds and written language in different parts of the brain. Patients can view words, such as "hippopotamus" typed on a piece of paper and find it on a flash card. When patients hear the word, they can't pick it out of a set of animal flash cards.[15]

WRITING TAKES WORDS, TOO

Writing takes on a different context when you don't know the words to speak. Nine months after my stroke, I started writing blogs again. I had difficulty finding the words to express my feelings. Getting the words to flow from my brain to my laptop proved to be even more challenging than I expected. It took hours for me to type out a two-paragraph post.

It's not that I couldn't recall the words, although sometimes I'd sit trying to think of a single word. When I had the right words to say, translating to the actual keyboard was difficult. My left hand was fine, but my right was like a lump of dead fish. Whenever I hooked into my memory and tried typing the word, my right hand didn't work. I didn't remember how to position my hands, so I could clearly and succinctly get my point across. My right hand got quickly out of position each time, so it was on the wrong keys repeatedly. It took hours to produce one simple 103-word blog, as I erased words that didn't fit and tried typing them again.

Neurosculpting: A Whole-Brain Approach to Heal Trauma, Rewrite Limiting Beliefs, and Find Wholeness tells us that capabilities destroyed during a stroke can be rebuilt in other sectors in the brain. The brain forecasts outcomes and likes order versus chaos. This capacity helps people concentrate on what's new while also doing something habitually. Once a stroke survivor knows the arrangement or sequence, practice makes it habitual. Then, it doesn't need to be relearned again.[16]

So many times, it was suggested I could use dictation software to type for me because it would work better than typing by hand. The funny thing is—I wanted to be able to type the way I did in the old days. I used to sit in a meeting and record it almost exactly as spoken. It took a lot of time and effort, but I can type reasonably well now. Dictation is an enhancement. I didn't want it to be a necessity.

What I've Learned

Neuroplasticity is a real thing. Last century, we learned that a traumatic event (i.e., stroke) can cause neurons to reorganize into different firing patterns. This news means the brain can relearn things lost. In other words, never give up. I believe that people with a "growth mindset" have a greater chance of recovery. They already believe they'll grow stronger over time. All it takes is effort . . . a lot of effort.

Some things can be impossible to do at first, but over time, the brain relearns. Interesting changes might occur, such as saying sounds and words differently. For example, I now say "S" differently than I did before the stroke, but it doesn't matter. I can say it well enough that people understand me.

TAKE ACTION

- Learn to speak again if you have aphasia, apraxia, or another language disorder. Speech therapists take the time to teach you pronunciation, words, grammar, and meaning. It takes a lot of effort, but I found that speech therapy was essential to my well-being. If you find that you're only partially healed, try a different therapy and don't give up.

- Give your home health therapists a chance. The speech therapist I worked with through home health care was one of the best professionals I encountered through my health crisis.

- Exercise your brain every day. Neuroplasticity takes time to develop. Working your brain every day reinforces what you're trying to learn and makes the new neural pathways more permanent.

- Understand how your ability to speak might be limited. I learned that the written word comes from a different part of the brain than the spoken word. I also learned that if you have trouble speaking, you have Broca's aphasia. Your writing might also be severely impaired. If you have Wernicke's aphasia, you have trouble translating, and although you don't have trouble speaking, it may come out as gibberish.

- Translating your words onto the keyboard can take time. Although you may know what you want to say, you may not know how to spell it. You may also have trouble keeping your hands in the right keyboard position. Keep at it. When you lose the words to communicate, a piece of you goes away.

Chapter 5

CREATING NEW PATHWAYS

When I started working with my first OT at Bull Run Memorial, I really didn't know what to make of it. I stood in front of the mirror and tried to brush my teeth. It didn't work very well. Combing my hair didn't go well either. I had to use my left hand to do all the things my right hand used to do. Think about using your nondominant hand for a day. How you eat, how you dress, how to tie your shoes, how to write—it's all different.

I could remember how to do everyday things, but I couldn't do them well. Getting food to my mouth wasn't hard because I'd learned to eat with my left hand in Norway. Keeping the food in my mouth turned out to be a whole different matter. I didn't eat much because I couldn't really taste anything. I had very few working taste buds. Most of the time, I swallowed okay. Jim stared at me while I ate. He was always wondering if I was going to choke. Thankfully, nothing went down wrong, but he was like a mother hen. Jim's mantra was, "Eat . . . Swallow . . . Breathe."

While I loved speech therapy, I dreaded occupational therapy with Evelyn. Even the most simple-looking exercises baffled me. One task involved a board filled with holes and a bunch of pegs. The only thing I had to do was fit the pegs into the holes. I struggled to pick up a peg.

I finally got one! Then, I needed to get it over the board. After some thinking, I realized I needed to turn the peg, so it was perpendicular to the hole. I couldn't get it right. I finally got the peg in after numerous tries. I wasn't finished, though. I had to do the next peg and the peg after that. I know the task sounds easy, but I worked up a sweat. I couldn't hover my right hand well enough to connect with turning the peg perpendicular. I knew what I wanted to do, but the muscles in my hand couldn't make a connection with my brain.

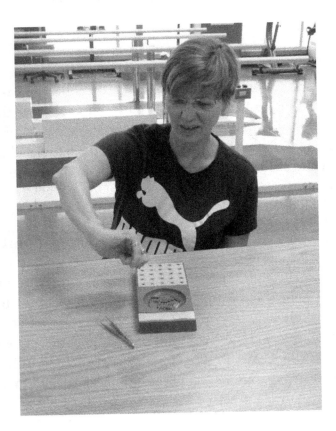

The exercises changed as I gained strength. A new exercise was done standing up and using my whole arm. The contraption I used stood about four feet wide and three feet deep. The goal was to grab the plastic shapes with my right hand on the right side of the arc. Next, I had to lift them across to the left side and release them when I hit the bottom of the arc. The movement would be simple for someone with a full range of motion. I didn't have that. Grasping was also something I needed to relearn.

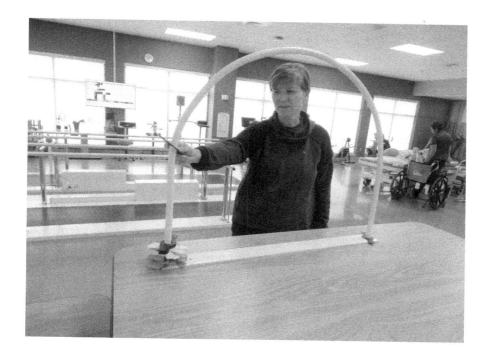

Once I finally got ahold of a piece, I'd start moving it up and over. I always got caught in the middle where my hand was supposed to swing over from abduction to adduction. I couldn't get my wrist to move properly. I moved a few plastic pieces over, but I made it happen mostly by sneaking pieces over with my left hand. I knew that I wasn't getting away with anything because Evelyn stood close by. She wanted me to attempt the movement several times, but she also wanted me to feel like I had accomplished something other than torture.

When I left Bull Run Memorial, Evelyn had the following to say in my chart:

> **Equipment special instructions:** You are independent with bathing, toileting, and dressing; however, you require supervision when gathering your clothing to put on. Stay seated while bathing for increased energy conservation and safety. You should use your cane anytime you're transferring on/off the toilet, and ambulating. USE YOUR RIGHT HAND AS MUCH AS POSSIBLE. Avoid the use of sharp knives in your kitchen, participate with meal preparation and light housekeeping as much as possible for increased development of right hand.
>
> **Toilet special instructions:** Use your cane!
>
> **Getting on and off the toilet:** You must have someone with you. See special instructions.
>
> **Getting in and out of the tub/shower:** You must have someone with you. See special instructions. (That didn't go over well with me!)
>
> **Tub/Shower special instructions:** Use your cane!
>
> **Driving:** Consult your physician about driving.
>
> **OT home progress:** Continue with your exercises provided to you during your stay.

CONTINUING WITH HOME CARE (APRIL 21 TO JUNE 5, 2014)

Terry came to visit me during home health care. She gave me clothespins that I had to open with my right hand. In the beginning, I couldn't do it with my third and fourth fingers. The index finger had the most strength, and that meant that I could open it a little bit. I could barely open the clothespin with my middle finger. Trying with either of the last two meant it took some time before I could get them to budge!

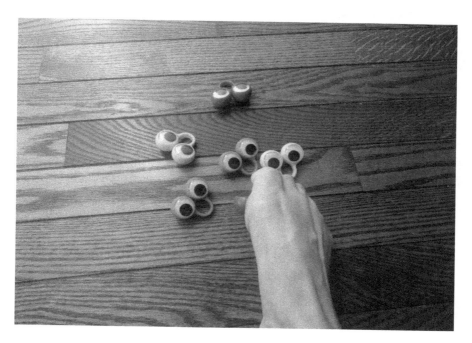

My right toes also didn't flex well. I wanted Jim to purchase marbles so that I could learn to pick them up with my toes. When Jim went to Target, he found "eyeballs" rather than marbles. They looked like the right size, so he picked them up instead. I actually liked the look of the eyes, and they worked as well as marbles. I could eventually pick them up with my toes.

Terry had me play with coins to improve my dexterity. I had to pick them all up and hold them in my hand. Then, I had to sort them by size. I laid them out on an "X" on a piece of computer paper—left to right, right to left. As my dexterity improved, she moved me down to rice. I spent part of my days sitting on the floor picking rice up and putting it in a bowl . . . piece by tiny piece.

Terry also made sure I got some exercise in the kitchen. Beating eggs in a bowl is much harder than it looks. Eggs should be beaten with a rounded stroke. My stroke had become flat. Even though I practiced, my egg beating still didn't have the round shape on the back side of the bowl. My knife skills needed some help, too.

Evelyn had been quite clear about staying away from sharp knives when I left Bull Run Memorial. Now, I had Terry telling me I needed to get used to using sharp knives again. Jim didn't like the thought of my peeling vegetables along with my fingers. He shopped online and found a pair of Basily Cut Resistant Gloves, with food grade level five protection. They worked wonderfully, especially when I cut vegetables on the mandolin. Nothing bit my fingers when I had my gloves on!

GETTING STRONGER (JULY 3 TO AUGUST 12, 2014)

I finally started therapy at Prosperity Hospital. Terry had been helpful; she kept me on track, and I exercised every day. My strength left much to be desired. Diane, the OT at Prosperity, was the first person to test the difference between my left and right hand using an analog hand dynamometer. The difference stunned me. It showed me how much practice I needed if I wanted to get my right hand moving as well as my left. Diane had me squeeze bright orange silly putty. "I. Mean. Squeeze. It!" Squeezing silly putty and clothespins started me on my way to gaining my strength back. It took a long time. Even today, my right hand is my nondominant hand.

There was one thing I was determined to accomplish in OT. I wanted to use my right arm when drying off after a shower. I wanted to be able to flip the towel behind me when I was drying off and swish it back and forth across my back. When my right hand and arm didn't work well, I had to think of other ways to dry my back. Eleven months passed before I could (kind of) flip the towel over my back, snag it

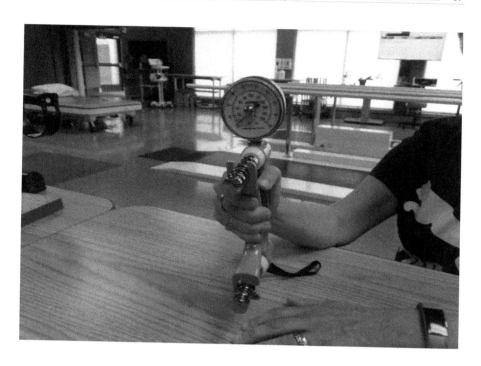

with my right hand, and get almost every drop of water. It felt great when I'd accomplished that small task!

TAKE ACTION

- Want to tie your shoes again? Occupational therapy helps you relearn the things you used to do, whether it's showering, cutting vegetables, or tying shoes. At home, I got up every day to go through my exercises. I didn't want to do them, but I knew I had to if I was going to get back the ability to shower, dress, and cook on my own.

- Understand how weak you are. I learned through the hand dynamometer how much strength I really had. I was shocked to learn that my right hand had become so weak. Yes, I knew it in one sense. But seeing my hand strength as a number was more meaningful to me because I had "hard" evidence.

- Learn to do the things you used to do without thinking. You can learn to do almost anything. As an example, I wanted to dry myself off after showering. Maybe you won't be able to do this activity the way you did before, but you should always try. The moment you stop trying is the moment you give up.

Chapter 6

MOVING AS A WHOLE PERSON

Physical therapy taxed me more than any other therapy. At Bull Run Memorial, when my therapist, Sandra, came to get me that first day, I felt scared and excited. Scared because I didn't know what to expect. Excited because I wanted to get out of my wheelchair.

Sandra took me to Bull Run Memorial's big break room. She stood me up and put a giant belt around my waist. We took off and slowly walked around the room. My foot dragged as I walked and stuck out to the right. I still walked like Igor in *Young Frankenstein*. Step, clop. Step, clop. Step, clop. I didn't look right or left, just straight ahead and toward my toes.

The right side hurt from my foot all the way to my hip as I walked. The most annoying pain was in the hip. It had kind of a scraping quality as I tried to move it forward. Before the stroke, I probably would have dubbed it five or six out of ten pain-wise. Post-stroke I had other things to worry about, like my shoulder, so the hip got a measly three or four. After walking around the room, I rested in my wheelchair.

After my short rest, Sandra loaded me on the arm bike, which looks like bicycle pedals except the pedals are moved by your hands. This machine worked out my upper body—and I despised it! The right side wanted to drop off the pedal. It took all my might to keep my right hand affixed to the lever. I kept rotating the pedals around and around. Finally, after five to seven minutes (all the while I thought of how my right hand toiled to keep up with my left), she released me from the contraption.

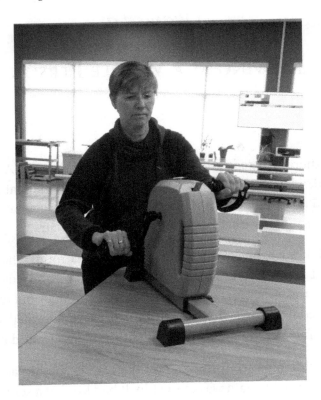

As I continued my physical therapy, Sandra required me to do more things. Climbing stairs proved a challenge for me. While going up and down the stairs was okay, I was challenged by the cane I needed for stability. Sometimes I'd forget to use it as I went downstairs. Sandra always reminded me to use my cane when I forgot.

Sandra also had me lifting one-pound weights. My right wrist, arm, and shoulder screamed bloody murder as I shakily moved the weight a little bit while my left side wondered why the weight felt so light.

When I left Bull Run Memorial, Sandra had this to say about my progress:

Safety and weight bearing: Follow safety instructions provided to you during your stay. You can bear full weight on your legs. See special instructions.

Safety and weight bearing special instructions: You must use your cane whenever walking. Have someone walk beside you at all times when walking.

Getting in and out of bed: You must have someone with you.

On level surfaces indoors: You must have someone with you.

On pavement outdoors: You must have someone with you.

On curbs: You must have someone with you.

Curbs special instructions: Use your cane. Going up: cane first, then strong leg, then weak leg. Going down: cane first, then weak leg, then strong leg. Keep your cane in your left hand going up and down.

On stairs: You must have someone with you.

Stairs special instructions: Going up: cane first, then strong leg, then weak leg. Going down: cane first, then weak leg, then strong leg.

PT home program: Continue with your exercises provided to you during your stay.

I couldn't wait to get rid of that cane! Clearly, Sandra wanted me to have it for stability. For that, I'm grateful. However, I felt like I had to get away from using the cane and use my own power to get around.

Sandra also believed that I'd sleep on the waterbed once I got home. I couldn't bear it! The discomfort of sleeping on the waterbed and the difficulty getting up resulted in me sleeping on an air mattress in the front room. I slept on the air mattress for months. I didn't care what anyone thought about this arrangement. It was more comfortable, and Pharaoh enjoyed sleeping with me. He didn't care where I slept as long as he was petted.

Continuing With Home Care (April 21 to June 5, 2014)

We'd heard from the people at Bull Run Memorial that stroke survivors who use home health physical therapists generally have less improvement than those who attend outpatient services. It wasn't long before we understood what they meant. Dudley came, but he stayed the least amount time, and he gave me exercises that I already knew. The only positive was that he gave me resistance bands. He also only signed the timecard intermittently, so I felt like he really didn't care.

When your physical therapist doesn't teach you anything new, you need a different therapist. Since the home care lasted six weeks, I ordered some CDs from Amazon including:

- *Discover Tai Chi for Balance and Mobility*
- *New Creation Tai Chi-Qigong: 7-Day Healing & Rejuvenation Plan*
- *Stronger Seniors® Core Fitness: Chair Exercise Pilates* program designed to strengthen the abdominals, lower back, and pelvic floor. Improve balance, posture, and proper breathing

I didn't care that I couldn't do all the exercises correctly. My right arm swung awkwardly. I could exercise every day with my virtual trainers.

Physical Therapists at Prosperity Hospital (July 5 to August 12, 2014)

Gratitude. That's what I felt when Jim arranged for outpatient therapy. I worked with Lori and Laurie at Prosperity Hospital. I loved the way they welcomed me into their care. They stretched me out on the table, and I felt relief as my muscles learned to elongate again. They started me (slowly) on the treadmill as I learned how to walk a little faster. (I started out at less than one mile an hour.) They balanced me on the Bosu trainer between two handrails and asked me to offset my weight between my right and left sides. I also had to balance on my left leg and my right leg as they counted out how long I could stand on each foot.

We went into the hall to practice correcting my foot drop by walking forward, backward, and sideways. Then they urged me to skip. I found skipping difficult because my right leg muscles didn't know how to propel me forward. Finally, they gave me several exercises to do every day at home. I did them faithfully. I wanted to get better.

"Foot drop describes the inability to raise the front part of the foot due to weakness or paralysis of the muscles that lift the foot. As a result, individuals with foot drop scuff their toes along the ground or bend their knees to lift their foot higher than usual to avoid the scuffing, which causes what is called a 'steppage' gait."[17]

No Longer Homebound!

The best thing about going to Prosperity Hospital meant I was no longer homebound. Jim and I could stop for burgers on the way home from therapy. Since I was no longer restricted to home care, I could walk outside and beg Jim to take me out for dinner any day I wanted. I asked a lot to go to Red Rooster. I meant Red Robin. I couldn't remember the name of the restaurant, but I knew where I wanted to go. Even though my taste buds didn't work well, at Red Robin, I could taste the hamburger and onion rings. I don't know why. We went there all the time. Poor Jim probably had trouble going time after time, but he took me a couple days a week or more.

The Women's Club (September 2014 to September 2015)

When I finished physical therapy at Prosperity Hospital, I was still far from being ready to regain my life. I continued walking very slowly. I couldn't walk backward much. I couldn't really skip at all because my muscles didn't remember how to do that on the right side. A "hop forward" on the right side turned out as a hop up and down. My right shoulder agonized every day, all day. I clearly needed more help.

I had been a previous member of The Women's Club, and recalled that they had an on-site physical therapist, Lyn Loy. I decided to consult with her to see if she could assist in my recovery.

A Note from Marcia

Almost 1,200 people per day need to have some type of support when walking after discharge from rehab. Three weeks after discharge, between 900 and 1,400 can walk without help from another person. Interestingly, every day, only 125 stroke victims in the United States can climb stairs and walk at a normal speed when they're discharged.

LYN'S PERSPECTIVE

I was really struck by Marcia's courage and energy. She wanted to get her life back. I wasn't daunted by the task because I knew that she was going to be an active participant in that journey. We were going to do it together as a team. The things that we'd qualify as deficits, maybe unstable gait, coordination that needed to be improved, or stamina and endurance balance training, were the components that I knew we needed to address. I felt totally comfortable that we'd be able to approach all those things.

The first thing that I noticed about Marcia was her determination. I was so inspired by that. It was clear this was going to be a partnership. It was a joy to have a patient who says, "I'm here to get to a better place." That attitude was her unapologetic way of saying, "This is me; this is where I've been. I'd like to get to a better place. I trust you."

I designed Marcia's program by listening to her tell me what was missing. Her input was important to consider in designing her program, because as I evaluated her clinical findings, it was important to customize a treatment program to address her unique needs.

According to Hindawi Stroke Research and Treatment:

- One-third of stroke survivors can walk without assistance seven days post-stroke;

- One-half to four-fifths of stroke survivors can walk without assistance after twenty-one days of hospital discharge;

- After six months, eighty-five percent of stroke survivors can walk without assistance;

- Seven percent can walk up slopes and stairs at a pace that would be considered normal by society.[18]

Early on, Marcia began practicing handwriting by tracing shapes to regain her fine motor coordination. She wanted to write a check and sign her name with a flourish. We had several things to work on that weren't defined by traditional physical therapy standards. Each time she came in, I'd interview her, reevaluate the treatment plan, and adjust it so it would be in alignment with what Marcia needed to get through her days.

On her down days, she'd cry. I remember thinking about how her authenticity was a gift to me as a healthcare provider. Marcia didn't have control over her emotions, and she didn't ever apologize for crying. Marcia taught me about dignity and being comfortable in her own skin. Yet, despite the emotions and crying, she was always upbeat about what was going to happen next. Marcia never closed any doors.

A Note from Marcia

Walking seems so easy until you have a stroke. My muscles seemed to fight each other and didn't function in a tripartite model (which is how the muscles in the leg work) to step and balance. Some stroke survivors choose safety over comfort, which means they choose to avoid walking outside where there are environmental conditions to contend with such as grass, pavement, sticks, stones, and sidewalks that go up and down. Falls are common. I fell, and it hurt. But I kept on going anyway.

Working with Lyn

What Lyn wrote about my crying is true. I still had no way to check my emotions—and she got them all. If having a stroke taught me anything, it's that it's helpful to get rid of the pretenses in your life.

If somebody doesn't fit with my sense of belonging, I can choose not to be with them. If you need to start something new, start it. There's only so much time we have on earth. I choose to make the best of it.

Lyn challenged me with a wide variety of movement experiences: coordination, agility, strength, flexibility, movement planning, and balance. I remember the first time I was on her balance beam. It was four-inches wide and two-inches tall, and I had to walk up and back while balancing on the beam. It was amazing how much energy I put into trying not to fall off it. I did floor exercises, walking exercises, and worked with weights that used my whole body. I did exercises on weight machines and against the wall to gain strength in my upper body. We tossed balls back and forth. Lyn told me that the left side showed the right side how to do it succinctly. The left side was the "big sister." It gave encouragement, experience, and practice to create "spillover" to the right side. We did a lot of cross-body work, crossing midline with the limbs to activate the brain. These treatment techniques helped the right because the left provided a mirror image that the brain could use as a helpmate to develop the skills of the non-involved side. Lyn worked hard to bring my body altogether, and I am grateful for that every single day.

I had some balance issues at first, especially when I rose from the floor. The times I fell, it came from other things, like a cat running under my leg. I could continue to step down (and hurt the cat) or I could fall. I probably would've fallen anyway if I'd stepped on the cat, but I wanted to relieve the cat of the pain of having this enormous person stepping on him.

TAKE ACTION

- Let go of what's holding you back. I had a cane, and it sucked. There's no better motivation than wanting and trying to walk without any help at all. This means you must get used to walking without your caregiver by your side, too.

- Find ways to exercise. Use CDs if the physical therapist leaves something to be desired. Workout CDs got me through the few weeks of home care.

- Restrictions sometimes don't make sense. By requiring me to stay at home during my care, we couldn't go out to eat. Since I didn't cook much, it was kind of a big deal for us.

- Make exercise a permanent part of your life. I'm lucky because we had resources to pay for an additional year of physical therapy after the insurance company deemed that I was "good enough." I now have a disability. Being able to move properly is vital to my continued health.

Chapter 7

REHABILITATING MY BODY

After my stroke, the left and right sides fought. The left side worked, as usual, but the right side seemed to argue all the time not only with the left side but with itself as well. The therapists all said to do my exercises every day. I did so religiously. Exercise is important for stroke survivors. It improved my memory and learning and kept me limber. When I slack up on my stretching or exercise routine, it takes me longer to earn my fitness back than it used to before my stroke.

Picking up the pieces of rice may seem trivial, but it took me a long time to be able to grasp one piece and move it to the bin. My muscles hurt and there wasn't any relief. The pain far eclipsed what I would've called a ten before my stroke. The pain wasn't going away any time soon, either. I not only needed to know how to deal with the short, choppy movements of my right shoulder, arm, wrist, hand, hip, knee, and foot but also to accept that pain would be my constant companion. I now had a different perspective on pain and how to suck it up and do the best I could. As long as I did my best, my sucked-up self would have to be enough for everyone around me.

Working Toward Harmony

Jim took me outside to walk for the first time on June 6, 2014. He slowed his pace and looked around for traffic as I looked down and haltingly plodded along. My right leg skewed to the right and barely lifted as I clumped forward. My hip ground painfully with every step. I knew that my right knee creaked as well, but I could only pay attention to so many pain points. It's not as if the pain vanished but was more like "that doesn't hurt as much as my hip, so I'll only focus on my hip."

The uneven terrain made for some interesting maneuvering, and obstacles filled the sidewalk. Where the sidewalk went up or down, Jim steadied me so that I could lurch through the unevenness. I needed to get used to the irregular and bumpy path. If I wanted to walk outside, then I needed to get used to dealing with whatever came my way.

I tended to veer toward the left as I walked, and I kept my head down. My left side worked without thinking. My right side took constant thought. "Look down and ahead. Lift your leg. Move it forward. Let it down." No thought when the left side moved. "Look down and ahead. Lift your leg. Move it forward. Let it down." My right arm didn't swing an inch.

The sun shone that day, and a strong breeze cooled us. The birds sang sweetly as we plodded around the neighborhood. I'd say that the squirrels were out, but I didn't notice. When we got home, I immediately went to sleep on my air mattress in the front room.

It took a couple of years to walk normally again. The thing is, I really don't walk like people who haven't had a stroke. Laypeople see someone with an ordinary walk. Health care providers see hesitation in my gait. My timing is a little off. I still have pain in my right foot, knee, and hip, but it's minimal nowadays. I have cramps in my right foot every day, all day. I still want to improve. It's a matter of figuring out what's needed to make improvement happen.

THE SHOULDER JOINS THE WORKOUT

It took several weeks before I began moving my right arm even a little bit when walking. It followed the same pattern as my walking. I needed to think about moving it all the time: forward, backward, forward, backward. The movement came back, but it was excruciating. I tried a lot of things to make it better, in addition to exercise.

I purchased a clavicle brace and posture support thinking that improving my posture would aid with balance and help with discomfort, but it didn't. Then, I bought a portable transcutaneous electrical nerve stimulation (TENS) unit, which stimulates muscles. I learned about the TENS unit from my chiropractor. It works by putting the muscle stimulation pads on the areas that need stimulating. Then, when the device is turned on, adjustments can be made as to how deeply you want your muscles to pulse. The pads deliver a small electrical shock to those muscles. The literature says TENS relaxes you. That's not exactly how I would describe it. I think my muscles were so out of whack, I didn't feel relaxed no matter what was done to them.

I combined the TENS therapy with a large lavender-scented heating pad. The warm feeling of snuggling relaxed me and brought some brief relief to my aching body. I still use the heating pad today. I guess I got used to the warm comfort, and now I don't want to give it up.

I also worked on procedures that my physical therapists recommended, especially in the shoulder area. Determined to achieve full flexibility, I stretched my arm behind my back consistently. It took a couple of years before I had full motion. Today, my left and right hands have the same reach! I admit that there is some pain, although I don't really think of it as pain anymore. I like to say that it is one-fourth on a scale of ten.

THE SNAP

I was so proud of myself on the day I snapped my fingers for the first time. It happened while Jim and I were walking. My gait had improved some, and I no longer thought about every step. I still walked with my head down most of the time to see where I needed to place my feet. I thought about my right hand a lot during those walks. It seemed small and useless as it dangled on the end of my arm. Needing to add a little spice to my day, I began trying to snap my fingers with my right hand. At first, there was nothing. The fingers could move, but there was no strength behind the movement. I tried day after day while we walked. Finally, it happened! I heard a whisper of sound. It took time, but eventually, I could snap with both hands. Now, if I could only get them to snap at an even pace.

NAPPING

During my recovery period, napping became my way of life. My body and brain needed to rest so they could recover from the injury. At first, I got up for short periods to do my workouts, eat, and read a bit. As time went on, I tried to spend more time out of bed. Sometimes, I felt so tired that I needed to sleep more than before. I felt like I was back at the beginning of my healing. I learned that those naps were necessary, just like when we're younger and experiencing a growth spurt. Each time I slept longer than before a new piece of me would come into focus. Because of this, I guess I believed that at some point I'd be the person I'd been before the stroke. My need for naps lasted nearly three years before I didn't require them every day. As my need for sleep decreased, I finally accepted who I had become.

BIKE RIDING

People say that you never forget how to ride a bike. I questioned that sentiment after my stroke. Determined to continue my healing process, I had my bicycle refurbished. Before that first ride (with supervision from Jim), I was overcome with uncertainty and fear. What if I fell? I only had summer clothing on with nothing to protect me from a fall.

At the base of our driveway, I tried to get on while Jim held the bike. It took some time because I couldn't get my right leg over the top bar. After trying a few times, my leg went over. I got myself settled and then focused on the next, harder part: riding. I was scared. I pushed down on the pedal and started moving forward deliberately. The handlebars shimmied back and forth. Sweat dripped down my back. I had little balance. I picked up speed anyway and pedaled up our slight hill. The going was tough because my right side didn't have much push. I got to the top of our slight incline and then did a wide turn in the cul-de-sac. The bike zigged and zagged around the curve, but I made it!

I rode downhill and the gravity pulled me forward. I went faster. (Well, it seemed fast to me.) The bike still felt precarious, but I gained a little confidence as I got to the bottom of the slope. Time to turn again. Another wide angle made the ability to turn on the bike possible. I went up and down the block again and again.

The sun beat down on me, and I was drenched in sweat. I called it a day after three times around the cul-de-sac. I needed to get off the bike. Trembling from exhaustion, I pulled my right leg over the bike's top bar. I was concerned I'd fall over, but I stood upright in the end. I was exhilarated, and I laughed happily at my accomplishment. I rode my bike! That was the start of many rides through the summer and autumn, and I didn't fall once.

MASSAGE THERAPY

After home care ended, I began massage therapy. I knew that the right therapist could help my broken body heal. I found Dolores. I told her I'd had a stroke and that I had agonizing pain (especially in the beginning). I looked for comfort while she worked my muscles, tendons, and ligaments and tried to get them in alignment and working together.

A NOTE FROM MARCIA

You must ask if there's a massage therapist available who specializes in stroke survivors. If not, then you must keep looking for a place that better fits your needs. I needed to find someone who would leave my neck and carotid artery alone.

These massages hurt. In the beginning, I could barely move the right side of my body, especially the arm and shoulder. Dolores worked on this area during every appointment. As I began to feel better, she'd spend more time on other parts of my body: my right foot, calf, thigh, and butt. Even when you're in agony, there's something special about being rubbed on the back without judgment. I needed someone who could give me that comfort while my body began to get better.

Dolores took the time to listen to my frame. She knew what my body needed. She'd stop, look at my arm and shoulder, and seemed to hear what my body had to say. I think it spoke better than my mouth. I asked Dolores if she would speak in my book, and she said, "No." She did share a thought that might help others.

When I met Dolores for the first time, she said that my aura looked like it was peeking out from under a rock. It was barely visible, small, dark, and muddy. As a person who didn't believe in auras before my stroke, I do now. Some people just seem to connect to other folks in a spiritual way.

"With strokes, the intent of massage is to stimulate the nerves in such a way that the nervous system can't ignore the stimulation. It's believed the tactile stimulation of 'Nerve Strokes' causes the nervous system to track and process the tactile sensations. In trying to find better more efficient ways of handling the information, the brain is forced to develop new circuitry by establishing cellular connections around the damaged areas... the primary focus of massage for strokes should be to stimulate the nerves."[19]

When Dolores moved away, I chose to get massages from people who worked for my acupuncturist. Each one had a distinct method, and they worked on my body much harder than Dolores had—at least, it felt that way. Maybe it felt that way because I'd gotten better over time.

While Dolores gave quiet, stress-free massages, the massages now were much more vigorous. I felt tired when the hour was over. I also learned from these massage therapists that rubbing magnesium oil, mixed with coconut oil, would help diminish the cramping feeling. Applying the oil has helped my right foot. It still cramps, but not as much.

TAKE ACTION

- Living with a disability sucks. For some of you, the pain will be a constant reminder of your stroke. Push through it and work to become as whole as possible.

- Know that some things you try will work and some won't. The clavicle brace turned out to be a dud for me. The TENS unit is something that I still use almost every night. You don't know whether something will help you until you try it.

- Celebrate both your large and small victories. I know it seems like such a small thing but learning to snap my fingers again was a big deal to me. It meant that I was gaining mobility and strength in my right hand again. Repetition and tenacity are necessary for the healing process.

- Nap when you need to. It may be that you can only get up for a short time. Let that be enough. Be sure to do something that will make you stronger while you're awake. Sometimes I went straight back to bed after taking a shower.

- Get a massage. It might hurt in the beginning. The muscles, fascia, and tendons might not know how to work in harmony, but it's important that they learn a new cellular connection through regenerated circuitry. It was years before my body started feeling good again.

Chapter 8

WALKING ON THE ALTERNATIVE SIDE

I've met many doctors since I had my stroke, and I've learned since then how to select doctors that are a good fit for me. The best place to start when looking for a new physician is through referrals from your friends and acquaintances. I also learned that other ways of looking at the human body—holistically—offers even more opportunities to explore healing modalities that might work well.

NEUROLOGISTS

A neurologist comes on board for every person who has a stroke. After I left Bull Run Memorial, I followed up with the neurologist I'd met earlier at Greensboro Hospital. He didn't impress me on the first outpatient appointment. He didn't seem all that inquisitive, although it's possible that I was the one who was out of sync. He asked me to recall three words during my first visit. After about five minutes, he asked me to list the three words he'd given me in any order. For the life of me, I couldn't remember even one word. I went back to him a few times, but we just didn't mesh well. I started looking for a neurologist who fit with me, and I found a terrific one. They're out there. You just have to look.

CHIROPRACTORS

Almost every neurologist has been quite specific about their advice regarding chiropractors: Don't use them—ever. I listened to that advice for a few months. The pain in my right shoulder wouldn't go away despite the physical therapy and massages. On a scale of one to ten, the pain in my right hip and foot fell a couple of notches below the pain in my shoulder, so I was pretty much ignoring them. The longer I let them go untreated, however, the more twisted I became.

I realized that the doctors I'd seen to this point didn't seem to look at me as a whole person. Instead, they looked at me from their specific area of interest. I needed doctors who saw me as a whole person and used healing modalities that helped everywhere, not just in certain places in my body. I would have been happy finding one doctor who saw me this way. Happily, I found three! And, all three were chiropractors.

- Dr. Fuller treated my food allergies and used acupuncture, starting in 2014. He later added neurofeedback to my treatments in 2017.
- Dr. Roberson treated the muscle system, fascial system, and dysfunctional movement patterns as well as relieved my chronic pain.
- Dr. Perih used Low-Level Laser Light Therapy (cold laser) to repair my brain's cellular structure.

So much for not seeing chiropractors.

ACUPUNCTURE AND FOOD SENSITIVITIES

Several friends had tried acupuncture for pain management, and all had experienced relief. I decided to give it a try. My friend, Rochele, suggested I try Dr. Brett Fuller. He has degrees in chiropractic, acupuncture, and nutrition, and, in her words, "does things a little differently." I made an appointment.

It was a crisp winter day when I saw him for the first time. I left home in plenty of time to get there early. Then Siri, my virtual assistant, couldn't find the office. Running out of time, I called the receptionist. She gave me directions. I was late by 10 minutes by the time I drove back. I was nervous already, and I had tardiness on top of it. Dr. Fuller simply took my lateness in stride.

As we sat in his office, he asked me several questions to understand my health history. Then he told me to sit back and relax, while he used the "AcuGraph" by touching a probe to my hands.

Dr. Fuller explained that this machine measures electrical skin resistance at representative acupuncture points. By using this tool, he can provide a more effective acupuncture treatment based on the objective and graphical representation of the meridians (the channels of energy) that influence my body's functions and healing properties. In other words, he could see the imbalances in my body based on the readings from the AcuGraph. Not surprisingly, I had several.

According to the AcuGraph, I had split meridians in the lungs, pericardium, heart, and gall bladder. Essentially, the energy on the left and right sides of my body had a "significant disturbance." That's probably to be expected because I had a stroke on the left side of my brain, and my right side had been incapacitated for months. My large intestine energy showed a chronic deficiency. I suspect it had been deficient for years because I always seemed to have constipation. The liver and bladder meridians were also out of sync.

DR. FULLER'S PERSPECTIVE

You can say I'm "holistic" (this word gets thrown around a lot in today's healthcare world and probably has many different meanings as those using the term), but I prefer the term integrative. My primary education is in chiropractic. In my practice, I incorporate principles of acupuncture, herbal medicine, homeopathy, functional laboratory testing, pulsed electromagnetic fields, and emotional healing.

I first met Marcia Moran, a quiet, reserved, red-haired, slender, fifty-three-year old who loves the color purple, which becomes obvious by her shoes, handbag, and clothing, on November 24, 2014. She presented herself to my office looking for assistance with issues correlating to the sequela (aka consequences) of a stroke earlier that year on March 30. Her symptom picture included chronic muscle pain, high blood pressure, back pain, TMJ (temporomandibular joint), low libido, allergies (to dogs and mold), along with speech delay, reduced ability to concentrate, coordination issues, memory problems, ataxia, and tinnitus (or ringing in the ear).

Marcia was taking Metoprolol for her blood pressure and aspirin as a prophylactic blood thinner. She also was taking daily coconut oil, probiotics, turmeric, and magnesium. She obviously had been doing some research on her own for stroke recovery.

> According to the National Ataxia Foundation, this uncommon disease imitates the symptoms of being intoxicated. Garbled words, lurching, slipping, and awkwardness are associated with deterioration of the cerebellum, which regulates motion.[20]

Ideally, with a stroke patient, treatment is always better sooner than later, with diminishing returns as hours turn to days, then weeks and months. Seeing Marcia some eight months after her stroke required setting some appropriate expectations, which she understood—maybe? She was determined to push certain boundaries if there was any possibility the treatments could make her better.

We added small amounts of DHA, alpha lipoid acid, resveratrol, D3, and methyl B12 to her current supplement regimen. We also added Nattokinase, an enzyme that "thins the blood"; L-Arginine, which converts into a chemical called nitric oxide that causes blood vessels to open wider for improved blood flow and reduced plaque buildup; and Hawthorn, which can help improve the amount of blood pumped out of the heart during contractions, widen the blood vessels, lower blood pressure, and relax blood vessels.

As I said before, treatment, including acupuncture is more effective post-stroke as close to the event as possible. Marcia received both conventional whole body and scalp acupuncture. The latter is more effective for stroke survivors. Acupuncture isn't just about putting in needles; benefits can be gained by how deep and how much manual stimulation is given during and after insertion of the needle. For example, the side of the body that's affected by the stroke will often be a lower temperature. By moving the needles in and out more on that side, I can elicit a warming effect. Various "protocol points" and "assessed points" were used. For the acupuncture literate, the common protocol points included PC6, SP6, LU5, GB20, ST6, SJ5, and LI4. Bioresonance, a noninvasive electrode therapy that rebalances energy wavelength frequencies, was utilized as well as electrodermal testing, used to measure her skin's electrical resistance, to determine additional treatment as needed.

During her acupuncture treatments, Marcia would lay her head in a ring that emitted Pulsed Electromagnetic Field (PEMF) for about fifteen minutes. Clinical reports show PEMF to be fast, safe, and clinically effective at reducing inflammation. While more research needs to be done, the FDA has approved PEMF for the treatment of nonunion fractures, urinary incontinence, and depression and anxiety among other conditions.

FOOD SENSITIVITIES AND INFLAMMATION

At the end of the year, Dr. Fuller did a comprehensive food sensitivity panel. I had food sensitivities to gluten, milk, eggs, and yeast as well as casein, some nuts, some fish and shellfish, spinach, and soy. No wonder my iron panels were so out of whack. I'd been eating a gluten-free diet, but I'd been eating spinach, eggs, cheese, oats, and gluten-free bread—all foods that I was sensitive to and that were creating inflammation in my body.

When Dr. Fuller gave me my results, I questioned them. He suggested that I try the foods on my "okay to eat" list and see how things went. So, I stopped by the grocery store on the way home. It took me a long time to shop because I had to read the ingredients on everything. I was surprised that many goods had ingredients I couldn't eat. Getting used to a new menu would take some time.

Sticking to this new way of eating wasn't easy. I longed for a piece of cheese or some bread. I was sensitive to milk, so everything in the dairy case was mostly off limits. Coconut milk was fine, but coconut yogurt wasn't for me. Coconut butter tasted like nothing, which didn't really matter because there wasn't anything to put "butter" on anyway.

DR. FULLER'S PERSPECTIVE

Reducing inflammation is always important for stroke prevention and recovery. Dietary modification is an important part of inflammation reduction. Marcia did have some food sensitivities with high Immunoglobulin G (IgG) levels to barley, casein, milk, cheeses, eggs, and wheat. She also had high Immunoglobulin E (IgE) levels to almond, barley, navy beans, corn, egg white, milk, soybean, and wheat. Avoiding those foods would be beneficial in reducing inflammatory reactions and help her goal of recovery and prevention.

Follow-up testing showed low levels of cardio C-reactive protein, homocysteine, and sedimentation rate; it appeared Marcia had been doing a great job of staying away from foods that caused inflammation.

EATING AND COOKING

IgG food sensitivities decreased my ability to fight off bacterial and viral infections. The IgE levels affected my lungs, skin, and mucous membranes. I'd been congested for years. While I'd been tested for allergies a few times, they were scratch tests, and they always came back negative. This experience reinforced my belief that you need to have the right doctor to address root causes.

I struggled to eat "right." I suppose having diminished taste buds helped in that I couldn't really complain about how things tasted. Jim didn't understand why I started eating differently. Then my chronic congestion went away and he came to realize what I ate truly impacted how I felt. Despite being a good cook before my stroke, now I cooked very little. I decided I needed to begin cooking again.

I began reading cookbooks. I found some ingredients could be sub-stituted, and I started baking, too. What I've learned is that there's a lot of hit and miss when it comes to cooking. We're still learning how to cook for one person who eats a gluten-free, egg-free, yeast-free, dairy-free diet, and the other person who eats everything. I've found a few recipes that work for baking, but many just taste awful. The exceptions are the gluten-free chocolate cake and carrot cake. Those tasted good even to my taste buds.

DR. FULLER'S PERSPECTIVE

My overall goals for Marcia's health was to create increased energy, reduce blood pressure and a corresponding reduced need for medica-tion, improved cognition and coordination, more even and deep breath-ing, and enhanced blood flow to the brain and possibly the left carotid.

Left Carotid Functionality

Although one neurologist said that my left carotid wouldn't carry blood anymore, it turns out he was wrong. When I had a CT scan the next year, it showed the left carotid artery had opened some. While it was carrying less blood than my right carotid artery, it still did some of the work. I don't know why it began working again.

If I have one thing to say, it's this. You must give yourself a chance to try different things. Doctors don't know everything. You must try a treatment or an exercise to get healthier, or your body will degrade. You may be the only one believing that you can do something. That's okay. It may take a long time. It may not work out the way you want. But if you don't believe you can do something, no one else will either.

A Note from Marcia

Sometimes you must put your old prejudices aside. I would never have gone to these terrific doctors before my stroke. Post-stroke, I was in such agony that I was willing to try something different, and it worked. It doesn't mean that I'm not careful with which doctors I see. If I don't like the doctor, I choose to see someone else.

Adjusting To Adjustments

I started seeing Dr. Oliver Roberson for chiropractic care. I'd heard about him from an acquaintance who told me he did micro adjustments rather than performing typical thrust manipulation. I scheduled my first appointment for Saturday, February 21, 2015. My only problem was that he practiced in Washington, D.C., so he was out of my driving range.

Dr. Roberson turned out to be quite different from any doctor I'd ever seen. He took x-rays of my spine and then walked me through them so that I understood what he planned to do. My cervical spine was out ten percent, so he thought it might be possible to relieve the tinnitus in my left ear.

Dr. Roberson adjusted my spine in an unfamiliar way. He'd put his fingers on pressure points and make tiny, incremental movements until the muscle relaxed and the pain went away. Then, he'd go to the next pressure point and do it again. Dr. Roberson doesn't believe in macro adjustments because they don't last long in his opinion. Instead, he determines where to put pressure to realign the spine subtlety. It works without any "cracking" along my back. I was exhausted after the adjustment, but I also felt much more alive. He treated me for several weeks and then put me on an every-six-weeks schedule.

Jim accompanied me on my first visit and watched quietly. Hearing the treatment plan from the doctor and seeing what it looked and sounded like made him feel better. Frankly, I was relieved. If Jim didn't like Dr. Roberson, I would've had a hard time seeing him. Although going into D.C. makes scheduling a bear, I think Dr. Roberson is special. He's one of those doctors who went into treatment to help people.

Because his treatment process is so different from traditional chiropractic manipulation, I asked Dr. Roberson to explain how he came to develop his process.

Dr. Roberson's Perspective

I've been asked by many of my patients to describe my method and/or style of treatment. I suppose I never really gave it much thought. In my mind, I was addressing whatever the body showed me was problematic. I know this sounds quite mystical, but the body has a language that can be understood if we pay close attention. Maybe I'm a bit of a body whisperer.

When I became a chiropractor, I believed the traditional manipulation that many chiropractors use addressed only about thirty percent of the patient's complaints. The muscle system, fascial system (the opaque connective tissue covering the muscles), and dysfunctional movement patterns (which are housed in the brain) weren't addressed using this traditional method. I believed that I needed to become an expert in the soft tissue that moves and supports the function of the joints, which are totally passive in movement. With a background in playing many sports, I knew the importance of performing at peak efficiency. I believed that everyone, whether an athlete or not, should be operating at an optimal level without restriction from tightness, stiffness, and dysfunctional movement.

Throughout my years of practice, I've taken what I've learned and created my own style of treatment. I started out the more traditional way, which teaches you to address the entire body and not focus on the area of pain. I've since learned that the area of pain may not be the actual source of the problem. In evaluating various areas of the body, my curiosity grew to learn more about upper cervical treatment for addressing the cervical spine. As with most things, the more one explores, the more one learns how complicated things can be. The cervical spine is intricately intertwined with everything in the immediate area. This includes temporal mandibular dysfunction disorders, headaches, and general neck pain. My studies turned to sports medicine as I believed this knowledge would give me a fuller picture of injuries and rehabilitation.

COLD LASER TREATMENTS

I was pleased with the progress I'd made seeing Dr. Roberson and Dr. Fuller, and I hadn't planned to see another chiropractor. Yet, I still struggled with aphasia.

In February 2016, I attended a Meetup group called the Northern Virginia Business Referral Roundtable. Each week, we were required to say our elevator speech. My aphasia made it choppy as I struggled to find the words. Most people don't understand how frustrating that neurological condition could be at times. Ron Wiersma understood perfectly.

He introduced himself after the meeting and told me he had a brain injury from a car accident. The aftereffects of the accident had left him feeling fuzzy. Ron had trouble connecting the words with what he wanted to say. He had visited a chiropractor who did cold laser treatment on his head, and it helped him feel more together. He suggested I consider this treatment provided by Dr. Theodore Perih.

I'd never heard of a laser used in chiropractic medicine. If it weren't for Ron's story, I probably wouldn't have believed a laser could make that much difference. There stood a seventy-four- year-old man saying laser treatments had changed his life.

From the outside, my aphasia didn't seem so bad. That's only because people listening to me talk didn't know that what I thought in my head and what I said aloud were two different things. In my mind, the thoughts were disjointed. I couldn't get my head around the discrepancy. If I could say the words I was thinking rather than the words that came out, I'd feel like a normal person. Of course, I wanted to try Dr. Perih's treatment!

On my first visit to see Dr. Perih, he spoke to me in the reception area. I told him about my problem and that I was nearly two years from the event. He thought Low Level Laser Light Therapy might help. We agreed to try a few sessions to see if I improved. These treatments weren't covered by insurance as the procedure is considered experimental. Feeling hopeful, I scheduled several sessions with his receptionist, Toneri.

Later that week, I went in for a treatment. Dr. Perih told me the therapy would last only a few minutes. I laid down on the red exam table.

The laser, about the size of a large smartphone, was held in place by a little portable grip. As he turned it on, Dr. Perih instructed me to do the cross crawl with my arms and legs.

The cross crawl is done on your back with your arms at your sides. As the left leg is brought into the chest, the right arm swings from where it rests to over your head. Once the arm and leg are back on the table, the process is repeated on the other side. I felt a little odd about doing the cross crawl. Up. Down. Up. Down. After a few minutes, though, I was finished.

The cross crawl is an integral part of laser therapy because it stimulates nerve cells on both sides of the brain. This makes the treatment more effective. While the therapy would work without the cross crawl, recipients wouldn't receive the maximum benefit. Even though I felt a little silly, I did the cross crawl every time because I wanted the maximum benefit.

After that first treatment, I noticed a difference as I went about my day. A small difference, perhaps, but a meaningful change in that the words came a little easier and more in the way I intended.

Dr. Perih uses Erchonia Corporation's 635 Low Level Laser Light Therapy laser because this company has done its homework. Approved by the FDA, 635 nanometers heals and repairs the cellular structure of our bodies. Other manufactures have a variance of plus/minus three to six nanometers, which makes them less effective.

After my first appointment, I dislocated my elbow and had to cancel my next appointment. I'd been training for a 5K race when I fell during one of my walk/runs outside. Jim took me to the emergency room, where they gave me morphine for the pain. I don't remember much about what happened except that the morphine corrected my aphasia! It felt weird speaking normally again. I was so disappointed when the morphine wore off and the aphasia kicked in again. My reaction to the morphine showed me there could be a way to get over aphasia. I didn't know if LED therapy was the answer, or if it would be something else. I needed more treatments to find out. I saw Dr. Perih the next week. My cross crawl didn't look dignified, but the cross crawl always looks a little undignified. I couldn't move my arm much, but we restarted my treatment.

Sometimes improvements seemed big, sometimes they were small. At the end of August, I went to my first ever seventy-two-hour Meetup to see how well I'd do in a chaotic environment. It ran the entire weekend. On Friday, I lasted from 9:00 a.m. to 5:00 p.m., although I was toast by about 3:00 p.m. I could barely utter a word. I went back at noon on Saturday, still not speaking well, and left before 5:00 p.m. Sunday, I strode in while they were doing presentations at noon. I probably stayed for only three hours. By that day, I was so tired that I could barely talk.

I was so discouraged by my performance that I told Dr. Perih about it. He needed to check with some other doctors he knew. Sure enough, he had a new protocol for me the next time I came in for treatment. I laid down and did the cross crawl as we completed the first protocol. Next, he unhooked the laser from the stand and held it while he did one-minute intervals on four areas of my head: both sides, forehead, and back (for which I had to sit up). This protocol, which focuses on general brain health, heals sick neurons. Interestingly, I found that it worked extremely well.

I was the first stroke survivor Dr. Perih treated. My case was interesting because I'd been dealing with it for two years. It was a chronic problem by that point. My body had healed itself to the best of its ability. We gambled on whether the laser could help. The time, money, and effort paid off brilliantly.

Dr. Perih's Perspective

Marcia's face was brighter than it was when she first came in. We see this a lot with pain patients, too. They're suffering all the time, and it takes a bodily taxation on them. She was brighter all around. And, of course, her speech was much better than when I first saw her. I know we've had a couple of setbacks here and there, but it's a lot better. Do I think this will take her all the way out of it? It may not.

Neurofeedback

Dr. Fuller piqued my interest in the summer of 2017 when he told me that his office was getting a neurofeedback machine, and he was going to California for training. I was interested because, while my speech had been getting better since I started Dr. Perih in 2016, I still had aphasia.

Despite having a better grasp on how to spell words, how they fit together in a sentence, and how those sentences should be uttered, the words I wanted to say still swirled around in my head. It bugged me that what I said differed from what I thought. I just couldn't get the words out of my mouth. I'd have to think of less precise words to say. That's how I communicated, and it was less clear cut than I wanted.

People who didn't know me before the stroke thought I spoke well unless I was frustrated by my inability to fully communicate or needed more sleep, at which point I couldn't utter a word. The folks who knew me before the stroke understood that my speech pattern had slowed since the stroke. No one knew how much I suffered. It was worth it to me to try to get rid of it completely.

Dr. Fuller invited me to investigate the IASIS Technologies Micro Current Neurofeedback (MCN) and learn more about the technology he would be using. What I read sounded fantastic. Apparently, MCN can help with many of the symptoms related to ADD/ADHD, addiction, anxiety, autism, dementia, depression, stroke, post-traumatic stress disorder, and much more. Most exciting was reading that MCN has been effective in helping mild/moderate traumatic brain injury (TBI) over eighty-five percent of the time, and the results are sustainable. In addition to the website, I read several books and did other online research on neurofeedback, and its predecessor, biofeedback.

"All the aforementioned conditions have a common denominator: The brain is "frozen" in a dysfunctional homeostasis that leads to dys-regulation. IASIS Micro Current Neurofeedback causes brief micro-stimulation to the brain that results in a temporary fluctuation in brainwaves. This temporary change allows the brain to reorganize itself. Thus, IASIS does not train the brain like traditional neurofeedback, but instead "disentrains" the brain by allowing it to reorganize itself and release itself from frozen, stuck patterns. This is analogous to rebooting a frozen computer."[21]

Dr. Fuller said we wouldn't know if MCN would help until I tried it. His patients who'd used MCN had received impressive results to date, and he thought I was a good candidate. Plus, I wouldn't get worse if I tried it. I was skeptical, but there seemed to be no downsides and a huge upside if it worked.

Dr. Fuller performed a Heart Rate Variability test, which evaluates the condition and function of the autonomic nervous system. The test assesses the effects on the beat to beat interval (R/R interval) comparing slow breathing, deep breathing, and breath holding. This test can identify abnormal neurological regulation that can affect healing rates and show levels of stress.

The test revealed I had a moderately increased level of stress. My sympathetic nervous system (the fight or flight part of the autonomic nervous system) was stuck or had a reduced ability to adapt. Dr. Fuller thought this made sense given the trauma of the stroke. I developed a kind of post-traumatic stress disorder.

With my test done, it was time for my first treatment. Dr. Fuller rubbed my face and neck with something that felt like a cat's tongue: wet, sticky, and rough. He explained that the skin needed to be cleaned and exfoliated to provide a smooth contact surface for the EEG leads that would be placed on my head and neck. No lotions. No sunscreen. The "gum" that he put on my skin needed a clear connection for the electrical circuit. He laughed a little as he put bobby pins in my hair to keep it out of the way, and then we got down to business.

Dr. Fuller placed five electrodes around my skull. He launched the IASIS device and we began. I didn't feel anything, but as we watched the screen, it showed my brainwaves. The application stopped, and Dr. Fuller moved the electrodes to a different area. We started the process again. By the time we finished, I felt good, euphoric even. I know that some people feel fatigued, spacey, wired, or anxious. I mostly felt giddy. After that first session, my aphasia diminished slightly. I eagerly made my next appointment.

IASIS doesn't treat disease, but it does help the brain to reorganize and reboot to a more normal brain pattern. While it didn't feel like anything was happening to me, clearly something material occurred in the background.

A Note from Marcia

I recommend you research MCN for yourself. While I can't explain why MCN assists in improving imbalances in brain wave patterns caused by stroke, TBI, memory disorders, or anxiety, I can say that it returned me to a more normal pattern of speaking.

After finishing sixteen sessions, I dramatically improved in both the physical and speech areas. My gait follows an even path when I'm walking. I no longer walk toward the left side of the sidewalk. Best of all, my aphasia is almost gone. I used to struggle to get the right words out, but now what I think about can leave my brain and come out of my mouth. I'm not scrambling for words most of the time. My aphasia makes an appearance now and then, so when I find words jostling in my head, it's time for an MCN refresher.

Dr. Fuller is always researching new treatments. When a new technique pans out, he'll try it. If he likes the results, he'll invest in the training so that he can offer the new treatment to his patients. Neurofeedback is one of those instances where I benefited. I'm grateful to Dr. Fuller and the IASIS MCN team for the courage to try new things.

So, that's how I wound up going to three chiropractors: Dr. Fuller, Dr. Roberson, and Dr. Perih. Each displays empathy, curiosity, and compassion as they worked through my issues.

A Note from Marcia

At a certain point, you must become your own advocate and be curious enough to investigate what goes on around you. It means not being afraid of looking weird or out of place when you try things. Sometimes I tried treatments and activities that, before the stroke, I would've never tried. After the stroke, I went into each activity or treatment with an open mind. As long as the activity (like riding my bike) wouldn't hurt me much if I fell off, I tried it. The same thing was true for learning how to communicate again. I looked to make speaking easier for the long-term, even though I knew it would be difficult in the short-term.

TAKE ACTION

- Like your doctor. You should know within seconds of the first meeting if this doctor has warmth and competence. You need to spend your time working with your doctor, not butting heads, or simply following what they say. Find a doctor who fits your style.

- Ask questions. It's important to ask about any medicine you've been prescribed and don't understand! I received medicine that nearly every stroke patient receives, even though my stroke was abnormal. After I left the rehab hospital and saw my general practitioner, we discussed my medications, and we agreed that one of them was unnecessary.

- Believe in yourself! Your healthcare providers may say you'll get better during the first six months to a year after your stroke. While that is true, you can continue improving as long as you think you can.

- Consider integrative medicine. Before my stroke, I never considered going to a holistic doctor. After my stroke, I became aware of a host of medical treatments that many neurologists, general practitioners, and other doctors don't even consider. I chose practitioners who treat the entire body, not just specific parts.

- Tell your doctor if you have disappointing results. They may be able to try something else.

- Look for answers on the internet but question everything. Do your research before embarking on an untested treatment.

Chapter 9

TRAVELING NEAR AND FAR

I have remarkable friends and family. On my road to recovery (which I'm still on), my friends and family accepted me regardless of how "with it" I seemed. If I'd stopped getting better, they'd still be there for me. Sometimes I still have a hard time wrapping my mind around that piece of information. I'm still learning to be grateful for the people who share my life.

The occasion of our wedding anniversary was the first time I would see many of my family and friends. That event reinforced what a great group of family and friends I have.

IRELAND AND SCOTLAND WILL HAVE TO WAIT

Jim and I have a tradition. Every thirteen years, we renew our wedding vows. We were going to go to Ireland for the big day in 2014, but my stroke derailed that plan. Because Jim couldn't take me to Ireland and Scotland to see castles or the Loch Ness monster, or gorge on pub food, he connected with two of my friends, Christina Molzahn and Donna. They agreed to arrange a vow renewal ceremony at one of the wineries in northern Virginia. Christina took the lead and arranged for the whole ceremony, including invitations, cake, and flowers. Jim didn't have to do a thing other than show up with me.

My sister, Dale, and her husband, Joel, flew in from the West Coast for the festivities. Dale took me to a salon in Reston, so I could have my hair done. After we arrived home, I talked my family into going to Red Rooster (instead of the correct name, Red Robin, because of my memory) for hamburgers. The weather was quite warm, and we enjoyed sitting around the table, chatting. I mostly listened. Having family around was healing for me.

Jim and I had decided to wear the clothes from our grooms' supper twenty-six years ago. Courtesy of the stroke, I'd lost enough weight to fit into the dress: navy blue with off-white leaves. I looked stunning when I wore it back then. Now, I thought it made me look kind of sad because women don't wear shoulder pads anymore. I really didn't care, though. I was going to see my friends soon, and that fired me up! I struggled to get my pantyhose on. After about ten minutes, I finally got them in place. I hoped I wouldn't need many bathroom breaks, given how difficult they were to maneuver. I walked out to see Jim in his light blue suit that has burgundy and white pinstripes. It made me cry. I felt truly blessed that I didn't die the day I had my stroke.

I was ready, except for my earrings. I'd bought a special pair and had planned to wear them for our anniversary in Ireland. After attempting to put them on for several minutes with no success, I asked Jim to try. No luck. I asked Dale, but she couldn't get them in my ears either. In the end, I had to give up, put on my sneakers, and go with the flow.

While I normally wouldn't wear sneakers with a dress, they were essential if I planned to walk around. I wore my purple pair because they looked better than the white ones. (I don't know if they really did look better, but that's what I told myself.) In solidarity, Jim wore black running shoes with his suit, so we were a "matched set." It looked odd, but we didn't care.

It had been raining all day. I'd hoped it would stop, but it was still coming down as we arrived at North Gate winery. I was glad I had my sneakers so that I could trudge through the wet mess. As I walked up, I saw my first guest, Josh Darrin, standing by the door. I didn't plan to cry, but it turns out I cried much of the day. This event was the first time I'd been able to see many of my friends. The love I felt for them seemed overwhelming.

When it came time for us to walk down the aisle, one of our favorite songs, *"Suddenly"* by Billy Ocean, began playing. I bawled as Jim walked and I plodded around the tables. I took turns laughing and sobbing as we renewed our vows. I was happy, so I didn't understand why the tears were in such abundance that day. Maybe I felt that I'd had a close call. Whatever caused the tears, Jim had a pack of tissues in his coat pocket and pulled a new one out whenever I needed it.

After the ceremony, we talked to our guests. I astonished everyone by not using my cane. Throughout the day, I either hooked myself to Jim or I made way from table to table. The day was exhausting, and I wasn't the kind of host I wanted to be. Some guests got very little of my attention. There were so many people talking that I shut down after a while.

Christina and Donna created so many special touches, many of which we still have at our home today. A collage of pictures from our wedding through special times, including trips to the Virgin Islands, Australia, Italy, Switzerland, England, and just being goofy with each other hangs in our bedroom. They also put together a picture frame by a bottle of wine that said, "Let's wish the happy couple another great twenty-six plus years!" It sat near a bottle of wine and people signed it so that we could remember this day.

The photographer Christina arranged made sure to take photos of everything, including some tasty goodies and a special cake. I'm forever grateful for the time and energy it took to bring this whole thing together.

Christina and Donna invited guests. These people had other important things to do on this rainy day in the middle of the week than to attend an event in the middle of nowhere. But they came to see us renew our vows. Our friend, Kurt Baumann, video recorded the event. I'm so glad I have that video to watch to see the love we shared that day with people we care deeply about.

To Idaho and Beyond

Jim and I agreed that we should see my family in 2014. After Mom died, my family got together every year to see Dad in North Dakota. Once he died, the family reunion ventured west to Montana, Idaho, or Washington. Jim and I couldn't afford to visit every year, so we saw my family every two or three years. After my stroke, we decided that 2014 was the year to travel to Idaho to see my family.

We left northern Virginia from National Airport. Jim carried both suitcases, and my job was to keep pace as he went down the escalator and through security. I didn't have my cane, so things moved fairly smoothly. At the gate, I was allowed to board first, which helped tremendously because I still didn't do well in crowded places. We settled into our seats early for the long ride to the West Coast.

Jim's Perspective

This trip was the first time Marcia had traveled since the stroke. I found myself watching every move or gesture she made. I'd been protective of Marcia before the stroke, but now I'd likely taken that to an annoying level.

I was still concerned about her eating and choking to death, even though that dangerous time in her recovery had passed. She still had to be careful how much she ate with each bite, so my body stiffened any time she coughed. My automatic response was, "Are you all right?" Hence, the annoying aspect that I'm sure she felt but never voiced.

I was also concerned about the hectic and busy aspects of an airport. Marcia could trip and fall, slip and fall, or get bowled over by a passenger in a hurry. Regardless, I tried to protect her as best I could. Happily, we had no incidents at any airports. In fact, kudos to the airline on which we traveled for letting us board early due to Marcia's condition.

When we arrived at Sea-Tac Airport, we met up with Dale and Joel who'd invited us to stay with them before and after our visit to Idaho. The sisters each wore a novelty hat that look like a crab and asked, "What are you doing here?" Their greeting showed normalcy had returned to this family, although the hug lasted a little longer than usual.

FAMILY TIME

Early that evening, Jim, Dale, Joel, and I went to dinner. The sun was shining brightly, and the Puget Sound rocked quietly with a few waves rolling in. The Cascade mountains were majestic. It was the perfect evening on the West Coast other than a seagull or two squawking. We had a fantastic dinner and then decided to take a walk along the pier. It felt great to be alive!

The next morning, we headed to Idaho. I still needed to sleep more than normal and dozed in and out as we wound our way through Washington. Eventually, we began a long descent into a valley. Suddenly, our Idaho destination was in sight, and it looked spectacular!

I guess I didn't know how emotional it would be to see my whole family. Although I was happy, all I could do was cry each time I saw someone new. Dale baked a huckleberry pie for dessert, a family favorite. Then, we picked cherries off the trees in the back yard. Yum! The fresh flavor of cherries rolled around on all of our tongues.

On Saturday, we drove into town. Before my stroke, I would've been in the shops looking to buy items for Christmas stocking stuffers. Now, I'd go into stores but have no passion for shopping. I simply wandered around behind everyone else.

In the afternoons, I took naps and did the workouts that had been given to me by my physical therapists. Later, I sat outside with family members and enjoyed basking in the sun, the warmth seeping into my bones. I drank wine, laughed, and watched people play games.

I liked being with my family, but I felt disconnected. It wasn't anything they did. Although I was slowly getting better, I didn't talk much, and I still got tired more easily than before. However, I was glad to be alive and enjoying the sights, smells, and laughter that comes from being with family. When it came time to leave, I found it difficult to say goodbye. There were more tears, a lot of them. Then, we were headed to Dale and Joel's beach house to relax and spend time with them for the remainder of the week.

Overall, this trip showed me that I could travel and survive—and so could Jim.

The Last in Her Generation

In September 2014, my aunt Esther died. She was the last in her generation of my family. She'd lived ninety-six years, the last few in a nursing home. She still had a sound mind, played cards like a card shark, and smiled most of the time.

Jim and I packed our bags and flew to North Dakota for the funeral. We met Dale in Grand Forks, and Jim drove the rental car to Grafton. When we entered the funeral home, it seemed people were everywhere. I was happy to see Keith and Jeanne so soon after our visit to Idaho. After a while, being surrounded by so many people began to get to me.

I was in sensory overload. With so many people talking and laughing, I couldn't keep conversations straight. I couldn't focus. The louder it got, the more shut down I became. It wasn't my first experience with sensory overload. It can occur for many reasons: a TV turned up too loud, a person's perfume, or overhead lighting, for example.

In my life at home, I didn't encounter this type of noise. With all the conversations going on around me, I could barely understand the person in front of me. I sidled up to Jim and my sister, and they comforted me. I wandered around the room with them. Eventually, we stood in front of the casket. Dale snuck two cards, a queen of hearts and a joker, inside the casket so that Esther could beat my dad at cards in heaven.

I would love to tell you about the church service the next day, but all I could do was cry. I cried because I missed Esther. I cried because of the music. I cried because I couldn't do anything else but cry. After lunch and a gravesite visit, we headed to my cousin Bev's house, where I again faced lots of noise and conversations.

I was quiet that afternoon. Grant Brandon, my cousin Diane's husband, asked if I was okay. I couldn't articulate what I felt. I was happy to be around people that I cared about, but I was shy about talking. My aphasia made it difficult to communicate, and so I shut down. If I could talk to Grant now, I would articulate how uncomfortable a crowd of people made me feel. My brain couldn't process so much information and my mechanism for dealing with overload was shutting down.

A Note from Marcia

When I experienced sensory overload I completely shut down. Thinking back, sometimes it was like giving up on myself. In hindsight, I would have done it differently.

TAKE ACTION

- Make sure to include some "fun" into your schedule. Even though we didn't go to Scotland and Ireland, Jim and my friends made sure that we had an anniversary party that we'd remember.

- Travel—assuming your doctor permits it. We decided to travel to see family and friends the first year after my stroke. It was amazing seeing them in person.

- Being indifferent is normal at first. You're not the same person as you were before the stroke. You'll either grow to like something again or learn to do new things.

- Step back from people when you have sensory overload. It's normal for stroke patients to be overwhelmed. You have the right to withdraw whether people understand or not.

Chapter 10

Declaring My Independence

Since my stroke, I'd lost the independence I'd known most of my life. In an instant, I became dependent on others. I'm filled with gratitude at those who took care of me (especially Jim). However, I needed to regain my independence; it was an important step toward my new normal.

Driving Topless

Loneliness—that's what you feel when you're unable to drive. We forget how connected we are until that part of you goes away. Part of me wanted to drive again because I felt so alone. The other part of me was terrified. What would happen if I got into an accident?

It was a lovely summer day in August when Jim suggested that we take my car for a ride to test things out. It had sat in the garage, untouched for almost five months. Nervously, I got in the car. Would I be able to maneuver with a manual transmission? When I sat down, I couldn't help but smile. Jim slid in next to me.

My 1997 Miata holds a special place in my heart. There was something about this particular car that called out to me, "Pick me! Pick me!" the day we bought it. Even after so much time, driving it still puts me in a very happy mood. The seats are a little ragged. The pedals are worn. When the top is down and the wind blows in my hair, it feels like magic.

The garage door opened, and the car gleamed as sunlight came streaming into the bay. I depressed the clutch nervously. I turned the key over and the engine roared to life. Now came the harder part—driving.

I tried to shift into reverse with my right hand. Ow! My arm didn't go back that far! I changed tactics and shifted into reverse with my left hand. I backed slowly out of the garage and onto the street. I worried I wouldn't have the strength in my right arm to shift. Turns out I was worried for nothing. My arm hurt, but I managed to shift every time. Reverse was the only gear I couldn't access with my right hand.

I drove down the street with the breeze blowing softly in my hair and the smell of freshly trimmed grass filling the air. I had a smile on my face again. Driving proved difficult, but not impossible. We went four miles that day. I was drained when we returned home.

I had to adhere to some driving rules Jim devised. I had to stay on city streets, no highways. I had to stay within a four-mile radius except for doctor appointments. Jim was worried about my driving, but he needed to get back to work full-time. I had to become independent.

I worried as well. While I felt the need to drive again, I thought about accidents quite a bit. What if I caused one? When I stopped at a corner, I looked both ways a couple of times before turning. When winter came, I drove the SUV because it had better traction. Even then, I still felt nervous.

It was three years before I felt totally comfortable driving the car again. Not that I told Jim. He worried about me anyway. I didn't need to make his anxiety worse.

CONTINUING MY LEARNING

I started my training with Personal Transformation and Courage Institute (PTCI) in 2012. It turned into one of the most amazing experiences in my life, and many of the class participants I met in the program still meet periodically for dinner. This deep connection can be attributed to the founders, Mary Elizabeth Lynch and Mark Thurston, who created a safe space for people to express themselves with wholehearted emotion and without worry.

I had a hard decision to make in the fall of 2014 as to whether or not I should continue my training. I felt like I had so little to offer because I was diminished in my ability to think, hear, and connect. I talked to Mary Elizabeth about my concerns, including my inability to catch everything said in a group. She encouraged me to come and told me that I could go upstairs and sleep any time I wanted to.

My friends, Rochele and Pat Carretta, had already signed up for Energy Awareness Training. With some reservation, I eventually did, too. Rochele came to pick me up that first weekend. I was thrilled to see her! As we drove away, I realized this was the first time I'd gone anywhere with someone other than Jim. It was freeing! I was growing into my own person again!

In the car, we talked like old friends. We parked, went in, and took off our shoes. Then the hugging began. I felt comforted, humbled, and at peace. Although I didn't know everyone there, I knew enough of them to feel at home as we started our day.

A lot of what PTCI teaches is listening to yourself for your truth. Sometimes you do the work yourself through self-reflection, journaling, and somatic exercises. Sometimes you pair up and work with a partner in the spirit of self-exploration and holding space for such exploration for your partner. There are also exercises that engage emotional intelligence as well as body wisdom that invite the participation of all members of the cohort group.

The courses focus on identifying your values and strengths and then understanding what holds you back from fully living your ideals and achieving your goals. The courses seek to give you the vision and courage to choose a different path and new way of being. The only barriers that you have are the impediments you bring to the party. You do a lot of listening to the other people in the group when it is not your turn to speak. The space is sacred and there is no judging. Confidentiality is central to this work and I honestly believe that the things that we share stay within this group of people.

Here's what I wrote in my iPad the first weekend:

> The trouble that I have with my stroke is really bothering me. I feel that I should be much further along than I am, be better prepared to take on life as I know it. It makes me feel sad, depressed, and question whether or not I'm going to make it. Will I be able to type? Will I be able to run? Will I be able to take on clients and deliver their expectations?
>
> When I look at others, they feel surprised that I am doing this well. It does make me pause and take a look at where I am. My right side is weak, but it's getting stronger. My physical therapist has given me exercises that will make the right side as strong as my left [in time]. In fact, I feel much stronger than I did four weeks ago. I ran for two minutes yesterday, and I felt great about it.
>
> I think looking from the outside in is an important way for me to see how far I've come. It helps me get out of my skin. Knowing that I would feel safe was key to my involvement

in PTCI. It came down to Mary Elizabeth, Rochele, Pat, and all the other participants. While I didn't feel whole, I felt good enough to make an effort. Perhaps that's one of the keys to getting better.

When noon rolled around, I ate quickly. I wanted to go to sleep so badly, and I did so every day. No one mocked me. When the class started up again, they called me. Occasionally, I took a nap in addition to the one I had at noon.

When we did meditations, breathing exercises, and dancing, I thought about what it had been like before the stroke and what it was like now. After the stroke, I felt sensations only on my left side. I danced and flowed a scarf around my body, but I felt awkward and tired. I was drained by the time the day finished. I looked forward to going home and getting into bed.

ROCHELE'S PERSPECTIVE

My friendship with Marcia began in 2012. For one of our courses at PTCI, we stayed at a state park in a wonderful cabin and walked to class every day. This experience deepened our connection and friendship. The next course was scheduled to begin after she'd had her stroke. I couldn't imagine being in the course without Marcia. It was selfish, but I believed that getting back to her circle of friends would be a way to help her come back.

Marcia agreed to participate in the four-month course, and I picked her up and brought her home each day. The first day, I noticed how uncomfortable I was in silence. So, I filled it with chatty superficial stuff sharing what was going on with me, asking questions and getting quick, short answers. I realized I didn't know how to be with the new Marcia. Things we had established, our close honesty, open communication, and boundaries needed to be reestablished. Should I talk about the stroke and path of recovery? Could I hold her frustration, sadness, and hope as well as my desire to hit reset and have this all go away?

As we went through the class, it was apparent Marcia the trailblazer was still there. It was almost as if the stroke had ripped Marcia down to her undeniable core spirit and that spirit was loud and clear and finding new ways of moving forward. Instead of using a pen and paper to write, she typed her notes on an iPad. When sharing around the circle, if she had nothing to share, she'd say just that. If she was tired, she'd take a nap. Just like pre-stroke Marcia, there was no peer pressure to be anything other than who she was. Marcia took care of herself and showed up with the same smile and open, honest intention as before. She may not have been able to verbally communicate everything, but it didn't matter. Her intent was obvious.

A Note from Marcia

I became aware of who I wanted to spend my time with after the stroke. I looked for people who I wanted to be with. I looked for people with a kind heart. I avoided people who could suck the energy right out of me. Life is precious, so it's important to make sure the people around you are precious as well.

Pat's Perspective

I'll never forget the joy I felt when Marcia walked into the room that first day. Even though the stroke had affected some physical aspects, and she struggled at times to express her thoughts, Marcia's soul or spirit was present. I could feel her profound courage, the power, and resiliency of her mind, her hopefulness, and her warmth. Her eyes radiated love and playfulness.

As the course progressed over four months, so too did Marcia. Each of us in the course benefited from her insights and her courageous vulnerability. I saw parts of myself in her and felt heartened and empowered.

Since 2014, Marcia and I have met periodically outside of the course. We meet over breakfast or lunch to talk about our journeys: the joys, surprises, and challenges. Each time I'd see Marcia, I would be impressed by her progress. On one occasion, I brought up a recent dream I'd had and discovered that Marcia hadn't had a dream or couldn't recall dreaming since her stroke. Through our PTCI courses, we'd learned that our unconscious mind speaks to us through our dreams; that everyone dreams but they often can't recall the dreams upon awakening. We wondered if Marcia's stroke could have affected her ability to slip into REM sleep, which is the stage of sleep where dreams occur. We also wondered if and when she'd regain her awareness of dreams. Such a day would be one to celebrate as another milestone in her journey.

For me, the most significant milestone has been Marcia's reengaging with her paintbrushes and finding delightful ways of expression through watercolor. As I listened to Marcia talk about her paintings, I saw a joyful and resilient friend who's an inspiration to me and others.

OUR FIRST FIGHT (POST-STROKE)

Believe it or not, it took me almost three years after my stroke before I truly became angry with Jim. I think that's pretty amazing. We'd just been to the post office, and Jim, who was driving, asked me to find directions to one of our favorite restaurants by bypassing major highways. I got out my phone and started typing in the restaurant's name.

Because I didn't have the answer quick enough for Jim, he started going the way he knew, which was the highway. I found it extremely annoying that he didn't give me enough time to search for an alternate route. I let him have it! Already in a foul mood, Jim gave it right back. My temper flared, and we got into our first argument since my stroke.

I couldn't believe that he didn't give me enough time to find a different route. He couldn't believe it took me so much time. We talked it over at the restaurant. He admitted that he felt angry because of my inability to react in time. He also said that he quite liked that I'd stood up for myself. It was hard to stay angry at Jim, especially since he was both angry and proud of me. I still lose my temper every now and then, but we let the little things slide.

TAKE ACTION

- Grab independence when you can. Being independent again provides a sense of normalcy. Jim had great concern about giving me power back when we went out to drive the first day in August. I gladly took it, even though I was still afraid of some things.

- Remember that people love you for who you are. If you have friends that leave, then find new friends. If someone didn't fit with my new style, I moved on to the next person.

Chapter 11

RECLAIMING MY PASSIONS

The first time it snowed I was giddy! I bundled up in my winter jacket and headed outside to luxuriate in the winter wonderland that had appeared overnight. The first thing I did was tilt my face toward the sky and put out my tongue to catch snowflakes. It made me laugh. When was the last time I had done anything so silly? I even got Jim to catch a few flakes as they slowly drifted down toward the ground.

I realized that I'd been missing out on the simple things that used to give me pleasure as a child. My stroke reignited my curiosity. So now every time it snows, I go out to catch snowflakes on my tongue and remind myself to look around in awe and be childlike in my discoveries.

BACK TO PAINTING

As the end of November rolled around, I knew I needed to get ready for the holidays. Usually, I sent a hand-painted card with cardinals to all my friends and family. I wasn't sure if I'd be able to paint one this year.

I found a picture that I wanted to try painting. It had the requisite cardinals sitting on a branch facing one another. I pulled out rough-grained cotton paper and began drawing. There was a deep pain in my shoulder that went down my arm. My sketching was not fluid like before. It was short and choppy. But I continued. It had become a quest.

I took a photo of the painting, uploaded it to my computer, and began writing our Christmas letter. I made several mistakes, such as missing prepositions, omitted articles, and misspellings. Even when I reread it, other than the misspelled words, the errors didn't stick out to me.

Just as if I were a child, I needed to learn to read and write again. Although I knew some words and phrases, I didn't connect all the nuances yet. It was a process. I knew that I could take chances knowing that I could be wrong and then try again. Or, I could disconnect and watch TV.

I chose self-acceptance. I was wrong about a lot of things in those days. I wasn't afraid to accept the risk because that's part of everyone's journey. My husband and friends would catch the mistakes, and I learned, over time, what the proper structure of a sentence sounded like. The Christmas card played one more role in my recovery. When I finished, Jim read and corrected the letter as he saw fit. Then I sent the card and letter out to be printed.

A Note from Marcia

Someone's ability to speak or not speak in my case is not a reflection of their intelligence. The person may think the same way they did before the stroke, but not be able to express themselves well, or at all. See if there are ways of doing things that better connect with them and helps them to express their thoughts. My outlet was painting.

Painting Classes

Painting before the stroke had been so relaxing. After the stroke not so much. Picking up and using a paintbrush hurt like the devil.

I had so little movement when I made a downward stroke with the brush. I decided to take painting classes in 2015 to see if I could learn to move my arm more fluidly. I looked online and found a class ten minutes away.

When I arrived at my class, I was met at the door by the instructor, Mrs. Lacrote, an older woman from South America who liked to dress in bright colors. She welcomed me with open arms. She had an impeccable studio. Books lined one wall. I saw four tables to paint or draw on, and canvases on five or six easels around the room. It smelled like drying paint. I'd arrived a little late, and six other women were already working on their paintings. Mrs. Lacrote introduced me to them, and they took a few minutes to get to know me. Next, she had me browse through some books until I saw something that interested me. I found a chicken.

Actually, it might have been a rooster. Mrs. Lacrote chose colored pencils for me to begin drawing. I am terrible at drawing. She showed me how to make my strokes stronger, but my strokes were still light. The head looked misshapen. Mrs. Lacrote showed me how to make it more symmetrical. I was proud of myself when I finished it. It slanted to the left and its head was still contorted. Plus, the skewed lines of the tail looked like a fox had mowed it down. It still looked like a chicken . . . or a rooster.

I chose a deer for my next project. Although my shoulder screamed bloody murder when I made the downward stroke in colored pencil, I could see changes in how I moved. The strokes had some arc in them, and the deeper colors showed that I'd pressed down harder. It took two months for me to finish the drawing.

Finally, I was able to paint using acrylics. I really don't like drawing, so using a paintbrush again felt great! I chose a waterside scene with a lighthouse. My strokes were still rough, but I liked how the paint flowed on the paintbrush. It took me two months to paint the seascape. I learned how to pigment the sky using red, white, and yellow as the primary colors mixed with white. I loved the blues of the water lapping on the shoreline.

Other than two birds and a cliff face that Mrs. Lacrote showed me how to do, I did the painting. It pleased me so much because it looked like a real painting. I gave the seascape to Dale for Christmas.

My last painting was a surprise for my husband's birthday. This one depicted one of my favorite birds, the heron, and was also done in acrylic. There used to be a single heron that flew over the pond near our house where I grew up. He fascinated me. He soared with wings outstretched, his long neck and legs extended like a pterodactyl. I painted the cattails green and gold to create a lovely background.

CHRISTMAS AT THE LAKE HOUSE

Since we'd bought the lake house, we'd spent almost every Christmas there. As we wound our way through the mountains for the Christmas holiday, I tried to feel connected to what I saw around me. Before my stroke, when we drove into McHenry and I saw the lake, I'd get excited about seeing the trees and the water. I couldn't wait to feel the inherent peacefulness. It had been almost nine months since my stroke, and I felt nothing.

We bought a tree from the local tree farm and then had a nice dinner at a restaurant we like. Then, it was home to put up the tree. Jim positioned the tree in its holder and put Christmas lights on it that night.

The next morning, I began to put ornaments on the tree. I dropped one. I used to get angry when I dropped things and they broke. I was like my mother—a perfectionist. This time, I reacted differently. I glued it together and hung it up on the tree. Yes, you could see it had been glued together. If you stepped back and looked at it on the tree, it looked fine. I realized that the little boo-boos in life really don't matter that much because it's just stuff. Maybe it's nice stuff, but in the end, it's something I could do without. It took two days to decorate the tree.

It smelled like the holidays in our house. Pinecones and cinnamon wafted up from the glass bowl on the coffee table. The Christmas tree smelled fresh and pitchy. I put the "candy cane" door ornament on our front door, and the bells jingled merrily as I secured it. The Christmas paintings and cross stitch went up while I put the usual watercolor paintings away. The Christmas nisse, Norwegian elves might be the best description, I'd been given by my friends in Norway hung by the front door. I hung the stockings on the fireplace and put stuffed animals out on the trunk. In only four days, Christmas would arrive.

And arrive it did. Christmas morning felt different to me. I understood what it was like to be truly grateful for life. With every package I opened, I thought more about the people who'd sent them to us. That's how it continues to be. When I think of Christmas, I think of gratitude for the people in my life.

I couldn't think at a higher level that year. Simple thoughts like my friends, family, buying and wrapping presents, getting the Christmas tree up, and working out completed my thought process.

TAKE ACTION

- Be silly. Sometimes we get so stuck in our heads that we forget about the small things.

- Look at things from a new perspective. I used to be really ticked off when I broke something. Now I simply decide whether I am going to fix it or throw it away. People spend too much time worrying about the little stuff.

Chapter 12

Finding My Voice

I'm an introvert. I've always been shy. Before the stroke, I'd overcome my shyness and enjoyed working with a team of people. After my stroke, I shut down again. In addition to apraxia and aphasia, which affected my ability to speak, the shyness had come back in full force. I worried that people I wanted to talk to wouldn't give me time to say what I was thinking. Worse, I worried I'd be unable to say anything. I worked on these problems in speech therapy, and I thought I had them licked. I was getting itchy to find a job so I could feel accomplished at something outside of myself.

Speaking to be Heard

By August 2015, I was fairly confident in my ability to speak. I began looking at jobs that I thought would really complement my abilities. I sent out four or five resumes and had a quick response from two employers. I had phone interviews scheduled for both positions in the same week. I couldn't believe it! I thought my life would be back on track in no time.

My first interview was with a corporation that dealt with hearing loss. Since I suffered from ringing in my ear since my stroke, I thought this would be the perfect place for me. I was so excited the day of my interview. I was nervous, too. I picked up the phone when it rang with trepidation. After we did introductions, they asked the first question. I couldn't say a word. They knew I'd had a stroke because I was upfront in my cover letter and during the initial introductions. The interviewers were nice and told me to take my time. So, tell me about yourself? Nothing came out of my mouth. I didn't know what to do, so I did nothing. Obviously, that ended the interview.

My confidence went from high before the interview to an incredible low. I was devastated by the time I hung up the phone. It hurt. I had the answers inside my head, but I couldn't communicate them in a way that made sense. The interviewers had no idea of what I could provide. The harder I pushed to get the answers out, the more elusive they became. My speech therapist had warned me that this would happen, and I hadn't listened. I needed to take a step back and figure out a new plan.

What was interesting about this experience is that I always liked interviewing, and I often used humor to set myself apart from the other candidates. Now I didn't know what to do. I certainly couldn't wing it anymore.

When Jim got home that night, I told him about the interview. He cheered me up. Since I had another interview scheduled for later that week, I decided to practice what I wanted to say. I reviewed my resume repeatedly. I swore that aphasia wouldn't sneak up on me. Nothing would prevent me from interviewing well!

Two days later, I had my second interview. This job would be with an association that needed a business plan writer. I knew this was the job for me. In the mid-1990s, I partnered with an entrepreneur, and in my two years with him, I wrote narratives for thirty-five business plans. Of those, thirty-three had been funded. I knew my results were impressive; I just needed to be sure that my answers told my story well. I psyched myself up for this interview.

When they called, we chatted for a minute or two. My answers seemed to be much better than during the first interview. When they asked questions, I rolled right into my answers. *Whew! This is going well*, I thought. Then, when we were halfway through the interview, the aphasia struck. There was no coming back. They asked a few questions more, but I was clearly not able to answer them. The interview was over.

I was heartbroken. I learned there's nothing more personal than being able to tell your story. When you're not able to tell it, it feels as if a piece of you is missing. I knew that I wanted to tell my stories in my head, but I couldn't say them. I knew I needed help.

CAREER-CONFIDENCE.ORG

Career-Confidence.org is a group of human resource professionals, headhunters, and recruiters who donate their time to help motivated job seekers find jobs quicker and for more money. I'd been to Career Confidence before when I wanted to switch gears in my career. I knew the founder, Robert Brandeau, also a stroke survivor, and thought the organization would give me the push I needed to get better. In January 2016, I attended my first meeting.

Halfway through the curriculum, we split up into groups. I went to a group that focused on marketing. We all introduced ourselves. Well, I tried to introduce myself. My voice was light and airy. I didn't express myself well. My thoughts and my words wouldn't connect. I spoke better than I had during my second interview, but the words were high-level. I couldn't dig into the nitty-gritty that swirled around my head; those details you must explain to get a job.

I went a few times, but I realized my stroke recovery needed to be complete before they could help me. I still needed to talk on the phone for an initial interview. The help they provided was from a recruiter's perspective on how to find a career, not a speech therapist's perspective on how to speak clearly and concisely. My speaking ability needed to be improved before anything else could happen.

NORTHERN VIRGINIA BUSINESS REFERRAL ROUNDTABLE

I still needed a group of people with whom I could practice speaking. I found a Meetup in my neighborhood called the Northern Virginia Business Referral Roundtable. They met for lunch every Tuesday, and I committed to going.

When I walked in, I was greeted by someone at the door who wound up giving me a hug. I don't typically like hugs from people I don't know, but for some reason, I must have really needed it. Interestingly, she didn't hug anyone else. As a group, we networked for a few minutes and then got down to business. First timers had to introduce themselves, explain what they do, and say how they found the group.

I had to speak in front of people I didn't know. Hopefully, I'd say something that made sense. The words came out slowly. I talked about having my stroke and needing a place to practice speaking. I was proud of myself for having the courage to stand up in front of them. With first-timer introductions done the crux of the meeting began. When it was over, I knew the Northern Virginia Business Referral Roundtable was different from any Meetup I'd been to before.

Coach Marvin Powell and Darren Marquardt founded this group in 2013. They saw a need for a place where people could get grounded, meet real people, talk through their issues, and gain a real respect for others. This group focuses on collaboration, communication, and encouragement. I had finally found a group that could help me. Here, I knew I'd found family.

TOASTMASTERS

In the fall of 2016, my friend, Donna, talked me into going to a Toastmasters International® meeting. My speech had improved, but I still had trouble speaking sometimes. Meetings were only an hour long, so I thought I'd give it a shot.

As we waited for the meeting to start, members introduced themselves to me. I also met the president, Marianne Meadows, who took me under her wing. Donna gave me a hug when she arrived. At noon, the meeting began. We said the Pledge of Allegiance and then turned off our phones. When I was introduced as the guest, I had a moment to speak. When I finished, they held their meeting. The meeting ended an hour later, and I'd seen enough to know I wanted to join.

The club had about fifteen members who attended that day. They had a cordial demeanor about them and kidded each other in a friendly way. I saw Toastmasters as a way to enhance my recovery. As long as I could stand up, possibly not speak because of my aphasia, and the Toastmasters could handle it, then I'd found another place where I could practice speaking. I could participate when I felt ready. I applied to join in October.

"Toastmasters International is a non-profit educational organization that teaches public speaking and leadership skills through a worldwide network of clubs. Headquartered in Englewood, Colorado, the organization's membership exceeds 357,000 in more than 16,600 clubs in 143 countries."[22]

They met weekly. I started slowly, doing small roles. In February, Donna recommended that I do my first speech during contest week. That way, I could participate in the contest but could skip having evaluations done. I decided to do it. I knew the group pretty well by then, so my aphasia might not hold me back.

I took time preparing my topic. The ice breaker, the first speech, runs four to six minutes. I'd seen others do slideshows, so I decided that would work for me as well. At first, my presentation was too long, so I shortened it. I practiced again. It was still too long. I shortened it again and decided to go with the flow. If I went over the six minutes because of my aphasia, I could live with it.

The day of my first speech arrived. I practiced a few more times and was ready to see how well I could do. I arrived early and checked in. After the Pledge of Allegiance, Donna stood up and gave the first speech of the day. I didn't hear much of what she had to say because I was too nervous. Donna finished, and we all clapped. Then, Marianne called my name.

Heart thumping, I slid my chair back, stood up, and approached the front of the room. My throat felt tight. I reminded myself to breathe. I spent time making sure the presentation slides worked. Then it was time to speak. The first sentence flowed! The second sentence started just fine and then zip—nothing came out of my mouth. My aphasia had set in. I told myself to breathe. I started the second sentence again. Halfway through the sentence, I seized up again. I was worried I'd completely shut down. I made it through that sentence on the sixth try. I finished my speech, shook Marianne's hand, and sat down.

I was proud of myself that I finished my speech that day. No, it wasn't the most eloquent. I finished it though! It was a start. It was a different experience than in the Northern Virginia Business Referral Roundtable. There, when I couldn't find the words, I'd sit down. I didn't ask for more time because I didn't feel right making them wait for me when there was a roomful of people waiting for their time to talk. The Toastmasters waited for me to finish my speech. Having photos in my presentation helped. I could look at them, get my bearings, and move forward.

TAKE ACTION

- Heartbreak happens. For me, it hurt the most when I couldn't tell my story succinctly. You must get up and try again. Maybe it takes confidence. Maybe it takes a new treatment. You must keep going despite the disappointment you feel in the moment.

- Don't give up. Ever. Sometimes things don't work out the way you plan. That's okay as long as you pick yourself up and try again. Maybe you try the same thing. Maybe you try something different. The point is that you keep going.

- Know when you're in the wrong place. It didn't take long for me to figure out I needed a different place than Career-Confidence.org. Trust your gut.

- Find groups in your area that can help you. As much as I hated Meetups, I know it was the right meeting for me to try. I was pleasantly surprised to discover that what I found fit my needs perfectly.

- Build confidence! Toastmasters International boosts your confidence. All members are there to learn. Everybody comes to the organization at a different place in their lives. You might be amazed at what this organization could do for you.

Chapter 13

VOLUNTEERING FOR GROWTH

If I could do anything differently, I'd have looked for more groups to be involved with from the start. My packet from Bull Run Memorial contained a flyer from Brain Injury Services (BIS). As my husband looked for rehab services right after my stroke, I guess they didn't have room to take me at that time. They fell off my radar. In September 2017, they were back on it.

I was introduced by my friend, Christina, to Michelle Thyen, the director of community and volunteer engagement at BIS. Christina was correct in thinking that Michelle and I would be interested in each other because of our shared passion for helping people with brain injuries.

Michelle and I had a quick phone chat. It was clear that I'd gone beyond the help they could provide, but I was intrigued by what BIS offered. Michelle suggested I volunteer for them. She sent me some links to explain what BIS does. I couldn't wait to meet her in person.

We arranged to meet for coffee. I told Michelle about my stroke, the challenges I'd faced, and what I'd done to overcome them, including participating in Toastmasters International. Michelle told me a little bit about what she did for her job and why she found it rewarding.

BIS supports many different initiatives, and I agreed to be a volunteer for the Speaker's Bureau. The speakers have all struggled with brain injuries from car accidents, gunshot wounds, stroke, and TBI. They work on preparing a script that runs eight to ten minutes long (with help), and then they practice speaking and refining what they have to say to an audience in the greater D.C. area. The first time I volunteered, the speakers blew me away with their messages. I had tears running down my face. It happened the second time as well.

My job was to help the speakers. If someone would go too long, I'd signal that their time was running short. If they needed assistance to their car, I'd help them find it. I was supposed to be a familiar face in the crowd for the speakers, too, although people with brain injuries don't always remember they've met me before.

I've also substituted for the receptionist when she went on vacation. The experience gave me confidence. At first, I felt a little funny answering the phone and putting callers through to extensions. The people didn't make a fuss if I got it wrong the first couple of times the phone rang. After that experience, I believed I could work in an office again.

A Note from Marcia

If you have had, or know of someone, who has had a brain injury and they need help, please look for a brain injury services provider in your area. It may be under a different name, so please look around online. Your hospital or rehab hospital might also have a stroke group that you can join. Finally, I encourage you to volunteer for your local stroke group. Many people need to learn that they can come back from a stroke. It's a journey every day. You might be surprised at what other brain injury survivors could teach you.

TAKE ACTION

- Volunteer. It will affect you in so many positive ways. I wasn't ready to find a job after my interviews, but volunteering at the front desk of BIS gave me renewed confidence in my abilities.

Closing Thought

Sometimes when disaster strikes, we don't get the chance to say things we always meant to say. I've come to believe it's better to say things now. Don't wait. I had no idea I meant so much to my nephew, Scott, or that my stroke would impact his life so much.

Scott's Perspective

I was shocked to hear Marcia had a stroke. She was of great comfort to me when my grandmother passed away, and I couldn't stop imagining the worst. How could this happen? She was too young, fit, and active to have a stroke. Now her life and Jim's life would be forever changed. I'm grateful Jim was there for her when it happened and have no doubt he's contributed greatly to her recovery.

For those first few months after her stroke happened, I couldn't help but reflect on my life. I knew I was putting things off for no good reason instead of deciding what was truly important to me and making plans to accomplish them. That fall, I went on safari in Africa. The next spring, I was in Botswana meeting wonderful people and experiencing something better than I could have ever imagined. I continue to live my life this way and am grateful Marcia's recovery has allowed her to remain an active and vibrant part of my life. Because of Marcia's stroke, I quit dreaming about the things I wanted to do "someday" and started doing them today.

A Note from Marcia

It turns out that my life taught Scott the same thing that my mother's life—and death—taught me. Live life every day as if it's your last. You never know when your time for adversity comes.

ACKNOWLEDGMENTS

This book wouldn't be possible without all the help I've received from doctors, friends, family, and especially my husband. In fact, I wouldn't be the same if their support had been different. So many times, you may hear about how someone has had a major brain injury and that person isn't the same.

I know I'm not the same as before the stroke, but I don't know what about me is different. Yes, I see the world differently. I'm more in touch with my feelings and tell those around me that I care about them. I know that my family and friends still care for me. They've seen me at my weakest. I had nowhere to go but up!

In particular, I'd like to thank:

My husband, Jim. My soulmate. He helped me through my struggles without batting an eye. He made me feel special—even in times when I definitely wasn't. He encouraged me, laughed with me, and always let me know that I just needed to try . . . everything. That encouragement kept me reaching out to try things, both new and old.

My sister, Dale Patience. She's the person I've looked up to with awe my entire life, and her husband, Joel. Dale and Joel took a break during the end of tax season to come visit and make sure I was all right and to support Jim. Dale and I have been texting almost every day since my time in Bull Run Memorial, and I believe we've become even closer friends. Do I still hold her with awe? You bet.

My awesome friend, Donna Hemmert. She teaches me how to be a better, more enriched person. We first worked together in the late 1990s, and it soon became clear that we'd be friends forever. Despite all the stroke took away, Donna has always given me hope and helped me gain confidence as I continued to progress. She helped me understand that, wherever I wound up on my journey, I would always be "just Marcia" to her. I love her like my sister. Thank you for the grit, girl!

Christina Molzohn, my remarkable friend, thinks outside the box and delivers stunning results. Among other things, she made it possible for Jim and I to have our twenty-sixth wedding anniversary with the friends and family who could make it on short notice. Despite a full schedule, Christina, working with Donna, created a spectacular anniversary party. She also hooked me up with Brain Injury Services, for which I'll be forever grateful.

Rochele Kadish, my amazing friend, reminds me about generosity, humility, and astuteness. She demonstrates these traits daily. Rochele helps me laugh at the mishaps that happen without leaving me feeling like I'm being laughed at. I admire her spirit, and I'm grateful that she decided to write what it's like when someone you love has a stroke.

Pat Carretta, my brilliant friend, shows great empathy, determination, and perseverance. It seems like nothing gets in her way. If Pat has a problem, she just figures out the best way to get around (or over) the issue. Those are qualities I admire and emulate. I'm appreciative that she found a way to talk about how my stroke made her feel.

Rebecca Kamen, my awe-inspiring friend, who reaches for the stars and taught me to do the same. You taught me to be childlike in my awe and wonder for the world. You also brought the spotlight out when I needed it most, and I am truly grateful for your insight.

Lyn Loy, my physical therapist, and now my friend. I think that people believe nobody wants to be seen crying in public. Yet, Lyn taught me (since I had no control over when my tears came) it's okay to cry. Tears are just a part of being human. Lyn is a brilliant physical therapist, and I'm grateful for the time she spent doing videos for my website in addition to teaching me about life in general.

Dr. Fuller, I am so glad we met! You took me seriously and kept my spirits high and uplifted when they could have easily gone the other way. You understand that your patients get better because you evolve the treatments you offer. Thank you for encouraging me to try neurofeedback. It has changed my life in countless ways.

Dr. Perih, your willingness to try your cold laser treatment on me, even though you weren't sure of the outcome, changed my life. You represent the compassion I believe all providers should have. Thank you for looking for a therapy that would work for me.

Dr. Roberson, my chiropractor who actually treats me for chiropractic care. When the neurologist told me that I couldn't have chiropractic treatments anymore, I was devastated. Thank you for giving me treatments that I feel great about.

To Keith, Jeanne, Shawn, Christy, Parker, Carson, and Scott. Thanks for giving me the courage to be myself. I don't tell you nearly enough how much I love you. I love you with all my heart.

Kathryn Britton, my writing coach at Theano Coaching LLC, who inspired me to finish writing my book. Your courage to tell me the truth about my writing made me create something that I am proud to share. Your deadlines also kept me on my toes. Thank you for your compassion, your humor, and being there when I needed you. I think you are the best in your business.

Diana M. Needham, my Business Book Shepherd. Thank you for showing me the way to get my book in the hands of those who need it. I couldn't have done this without your help!

Lisbeth Tanz, at Fuzzy Dog, LLC, for agreeing to edit my book. You had so many questions before the editing process started, and I'm so grateful for how you gently showed me that I still needed help. You made this book ready for prime time.

Appendix

Brain Injury Services

BIS supplies the care people need, not only to get better physically but emotionally. They offer support groups to caregivers as well. That's so important because taking care of someone with a brain injury is challenging. Even more impressive is that their services are free. They offer:

- Adult Case Management to capture the intricate needs of survivors who have experienced disabilities in cognition, behavior, and physical action. The goal? Maximize clients' strengths and abilities and create links to the community.

- Pediatric Case Management, which includes education, recreation, vocation, medical services and rehabilitation, emotional supports, strategies for managing life, transition to adulthood, benefit programs, and independence. BIS also creates fun activities for the people who care about these children.

- ADAPT Clubhouse, a work-ordered day so people with brain injuries can experience rewarding lives through skill building, volunteerism, vocational exploration, and Employment Development Services (EDS).

- Counseling Services focuses on helping confront emotional uses for people with brain injuries and family members.

- ComPASS: (Community Participation And Skill-building Services) Department consists of committed occupational therapists who aid people with brain injuries develop cognitive rehabilitation, assistive technology, and other therapeutic approaches.

- Veterans Integration Program contains resources, education or advocacy for all branches of service. They encourage networking with other survivors of brain injuries, assistive technology consultation, counseling referrals, and training to name a few.

- Vocational Services takes employment seriously. It is a major milestone for brain injury survivors to find a job. Employment means autonomy, dignity, and reintegration into society. Finding (and keeping) a job can be a challenge because employers might not understand what they need. The brain injury survivor might not know what s/he needs either.

- Volunteer Programs:
  o Speakers Bureau participants tell their stories to let the members of the community know how their lives have been changed. They inspire those in nursing homes, universities, rehab centers, and hospitals. BIS helps survivors to craft their stories, practice, and introduce them to the various venues to share what happened.
  o PALS (Providing a Link For Survivors) provides a friendship between a brain injury survivor and a volunteer for a year (or more). It is just one more way that they help regain their social skills in society.
  o Person-centered volunteering also creates friendships that focus on the brain injury survivors' goals, which the client cannot do alone.

- Groups that give brain injury survivors, caregivers, and families a place to talk and learn. They include: Caregiver's Group,

Loudoun County TBI Support Group, Loudoun County Women's Lunch Bunch, Recovery Group, Women's Coffee Support Group, Women's Lunch Bunch, and Women's Lunch Bunch.

- Community Outreach constantly sees opportunities to engage with and support other professionals and community resources who are involved in serving survivors of brain injury.

I want to thank Michelle Thyen and the rest of those who give so much to this very special group of people. Your help makes brain injury survivors realize that, while each one of us is on our own special journey, we are not alone.

References

1. "Stroke," NIH Fact Sheet, https://report.nih.gov/NIHfactsheets/ViewFactSheet.aspx?csid=117.

2. Anahad O'Connor, "Garbled Texting as a Sign of Stroke," *Well* (blog), *New York Times*, March 9, 2013, https://well.blogs.nytimes.com/2013/03/19/garbled-texting-as-a-sign-of-stroke/.

3. "Stroke," National Heart, Lung, and Blood Institute, https://www.nhlbi.nih.gov/health-topics/stroke.

4. "Hemorrhagic transformation of ischemic stroke," Medlink Neurology, http://www.medlink.com/article/hemorrhagic_transformation_of_ischemic_stroke.

5. "What is the Difference between a Stroke and an Aneurysm?" (blog), FlintRehab, September 17, 2018, https://www.flintrehab.com/2018/stroke-vs-aneurysm-difference/.

6. Sandra Deane, MD, Michael A. Gil, PA-C, Francis L. Counselman, MD, "A Spontaneous Internal Carotid Artery Dissection Presenting with Headache and Miosis," *Emergency Medicine* (blog), MDEdge, July 2016, https://www.mdedge.com/emergencymedicine/article/110156/spontaneous-internal-carotid-artery-dissection-presenting-headache

7. "9 Facts about Stroke Patients and Dysphagia," (blog), Thick-It, June 25, 2014, https://thickit.com/9-facts-about-stroke-patients-and-dysphagia/.

8. Grethe Andersen, "Treatment of Uncontrolled Crying after Stroke," *ResearchGate,* March 1995, https://www.researchgate.net/publication/15488542_Treatment_of_Uncontrolled_Crying_After_Stroke.

9. "Aphasia," Health, National Institute on Deafness and Other Communication Disorders, December 2015, https://www.nidcd.nih.gov/health/aphasia.

10. "Apraxia of Speech," Health, National Institute on Deafness and Other Communication Disorders, September 2016, https://www.nidcd.nih.gov/health/apraxia-speech.

11. "Arterial Dissection," Neurology and Neurosurgery, Johns Hopkins Medicine, https://www.hopkinsmedicine.org/neurology_neurosurgery/centers_clinics/pediatric_neurovascular/conditions/arterial%20dissection.html.

12. "Anomic Aphasia," Wikimedia Foundation, last modified May 2, 2019, 15:28, https://en.wikipedia.org/wiki/Anomic_aphasia.

13. "Cognitive Impairment and Memory Dysfunction after a Stroke Diagnosis: a Post-stroke Memory Assessment," Neuropsychhiatric Disease and Treatment, September 4, 2014, https://www.ncbi.nlm.nih.gov/pmc/articles/PMC4164290/.

14. "Broca's Area vs. Wernicke's Area," Askwonder, https://askwonder.com/q/brocas-area-vs-wernickes-area-55392b58ed1d710800d80a00.

15. Kristin Samuelson, "Brain Region Discovered that Processes Only Spoken, Not Written Words," Northwestern Now, March 21, 2019, https://news.northwestern.edu/stories/2019/03/ppa-visual-auditory/.

16. Lisa Wimberger, *Neurosculpting: A Whole-Brain Approach to Heal Trauma, Rewrite Limiting Beliefs, and Find Wholeness* (Boulder: Sounds True, Inc., 2014), Pages 9-10.

17. "Foot Drop Information Page," National Institute of Neurological Disorders and Stroke, March 2019, https://www.ninds.nih.gov/Disorders/All-Disorders/Foot-Drop-Information-Page.

18. Chitralakshmi K. Balasubramanian, David J. Clark, and Emily J. Fox, "Walking Adaptability after a Stroke and Its Assessment in Clinical Settings," Stroke Research and Treatment, Hindawi, http://dx.doi.org/10.1155/2014/591013.

19. John P. Cartmell, LMP, "Massage for Strokes," Diet Advisor, http://www.dietadvisor.com/papers_letters_strokes.htm.

20. "What is Ataxia?" National Ataxia Foundation, https://ataxia.org/what-is-ataxia/.

21. "Stroke and Micro Current Neurofeedback," IASIS Technologies, https://microcurrentneurofeedback.com/stroke-help-neurofeedback/.

22. "What is Toastmasters?" Toastmasters International, https://www.toastmasters.org/about/all-about-toastmasters.

About the Author

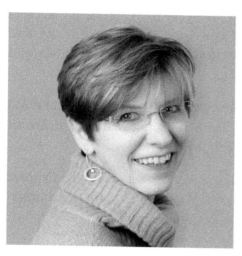

Marcia Moran has written over fifty business plans and helped entrepreneurs strategize over how to differentiate their companies in changing environments. Her twenty-plus years of experience helping other entrepreneurs encouraged her to found her own firm, Performance Architect, in 2012 and co-founded Positive Business DC that same year.

After suffering a major stroke in 2014, Marcia applied her skills in planning and strategy as she strived to become whole. She joined Toastmasters International© hoping to regain her speaking abilities. Two years later she pushed beyond her comfort zone to become a club officer in 2017, then Area Director in 2019.

A woman of many talents, she attended Skirinssal Folkehoyskole in Sandefjord, Norway and studied art. She also earned a certificate in Well-being Foundations of Personal Transformation from the Personal Transformation and Courage Institute in Virginia. She volunteers at Brain Injury Services, supporting their Speakers Bureau program.

Marcia created *Stroke Forward* because she felt there is a need to share hope to stroke survivors and their caregivers. Learning to become her own health advocate one step a time and exploring holistic methods for healing are keys to her recovery. Marcia speaks and shares her message of hope, inspiration, healing, and a way forward as she goes across the country. She welcomes new opportunities to help both individuals and organizations affected by major health crises move forward.

Marcia lives with her husband Jim, two very loud cats, and two birds near Washington, DC. Jim played a role of caregiver, advocate, and played a pivotal role in *Stroke* **FORWARD**. His observations and experiences are captured in the book.

On weekends, Marcia, Jim, and the cats go to Deep Creek, Maryland where Marcia paints watercolors. In the evening Marcia and Jim sit out on the deck and watch fireflies flit by.

Marcia holds a B.S. in Political Science with a magna cum laude from the University of North Dakota and a Master's in Business Administration, from Chapman University, in California.

Visit https://www.strokeforward.com/ for more information.

Connect with Marcia on social media.

- https://www.linkedin.com/in/marciamoran/
- https://www.facebook.com/StrokeForward/
- @Stroke_Forward

A Special Bonus from Marcia

Now that you've read *Stroke* **FORWARD,** you are on your way to overcoming the hurdles of dealing with a brain injury. Plus, you have received insights from my story about how we "took action," so you can start applying the lessons that we had to learn on the fly and many times, the hard way.

There's so much confusing information out there about strokes and brain injuries. I learned from reading a number of books, blog posts, and videos as I struggled to find out how to get "whole." The wisdom gained along the way is shared here in the hope it will help you. As you finish this book, you're armed with more information to keep moving forward. With hard work and perseverance to build new neuropathways, you can make a difference in your life regardless of how the stroke impacted you.

I've created a special bonus gift, just for you. It's your *Stroke Forward Toolkit*, which is a compilation of different exercise videos, my recommended resource list, and a guide with my favorite lessons, the ones that had the greatest impact in my recovery. While the exercise videos are offered for sale, you can claim them (and the rest of the goodies) for free here: **https://www.strokeforward.com/bookbonus**. As an additional bonus, you will receive more tips and information to help you on this journey. You may, of course, unsubscribe at any time.

The sooner you discover how to gain strength and confidence and learn ways to overcome the heartbreak, the better your chances for gaining your life back. It is, after all, a numbers game. Although you can get better every day, week, month, or even years later, the sooner you start the journey, the more progress you will make.

I'm in your corner. Let me know if I can help further.

Here's to being a thriving stroke survivor!

All my best,

CPSIA information can be obtained
at www.ICGtesting.com
Printed in the USA
FFHW012153291019
55844692-61737FF

9 781733 258708